Guide to Professional Development in Compliance

Jan C. Heller, PhD
System Director
Office of Ethics and Theology
Providence Health System
Seattle, Washington

Joseph E. Murphy
Partner
Compliance Systems Legal Group
Managing Director
Integrity Interactive Corporation
Haddonfield, New Jersey

Mark E. Meaney, PhD
Vice President of Programs and Publications/
Health Care Ethicist
Midwest Bioethics Center
Kansas City, Missouri

AN ASPEN PUBLICATION®
Aspen Publishers, Inc.
Gaithersburg, Maryland
2001

Library of Congress Cataloging-in-Publication Data

Heller, Jan Christian.
Guide to professional development in compliance/Jan C. Heller,
Mark E. Meaney, Joseph E. Murphy.
p. cm.
Includes bibliographical references and index.
ISBN 0-8342-1874-7
1. Medical care—Standards—United States.
2. Compliance auditing—United States.
I. Meaney, Mark E. II. Murphy, Joseph E., 1948– III. Title.
RA399.A3 H45 2001
362.1'02'1873—dc21
2001018862

About Aspen Publishers • For more than 40 years, Aspen has been a leading professional publisher in a variety of disciplines. Aspen's vast information resources are available in both print and electronic formats. We are committed to providing the highest quality information available in the most appropriate format for our customers. Visit Aspen's Internet site for more information resources, directories, articles, and a searchable version of Aspen's full catalog, including the most recent publications: **www.aspenpublishers.com**
Aspen Publishers, Inc. • The hallmark of quality in publishing
Member of the worldwide Wolters Kluwer group

Editorial Services: Nora McElfish
Library of Congress Catalog Card Number: 2001018862
ISBN: 0-8342-1874-7

Printed in the United States of America

1 2 3 4 5

Contents

iii

Contributors

Anne Adams, JD, MS
Chief Compliance Officer
Emory Healthcare, Inc.
Emory Medical Care Foundation
Decatur, Georgia

Mary Ann Bowman Beil, MTS
Corporate Ethics and Compliance
    Officer
Memorial Health
Savannah, Georgia

Randal J. Dennings, BA, LLB
(Hons)
Partner
Clayton Utz Lawyers
Brisbane, Australia

John R. Guetter, PhD
Clinical and Consulting
    Psychologist
Manheim, Pennsylvania

Jan C. Heller, PhD
System Director
Office of Ethics and Theology
Providence Health System
Seattle, Washington
jheller2@providence.org

George Khushf, PhD
Humanities Director
Center for Bioethics
Institute of Public Affairs
University of South Carolina
Columbia, South Carolina

Felicia McAleer, SPHR
Founding Partner
The McAleer Group, Inc.
Partner
CEO International, Inc.
Woodstock, Georgia

Mark E. Meaney, PhD
Vice President of Programs and
   Publications/Health Care
   Ethicist
Midwest Bioethics Center
Kansas City, Missouri
mmeaney@midbio.org

Joseph E. Murphy
Partner
Compliance Systems Legal Group
Managing Director
Integrity Interactive Corporation
Haddonfield, New Jersey
jemurphy@cslg.com

Christine Parker, BA, LLB, PhD
Senior Lecturer
Law Faculty
University of New South Wales
Sydney, Australia

Winthrop M. Swenson
Partner
Compliance Systems Legal Group
Takoma Park, Maryland

Preface

The U.S. federal government is focusing unprecedented levels of attention and effort on encouraging the establishment of voluntary corporate compliance programs. After the U.S. Sentencing Commission wrote the Organizational Sentencing Guidelines into law in 1991, partly in response to its efforts to bring the defense and paper product industries into compliance, the federal government has more recently turned its attention to health care. In doing so, it has strengthened the False Claims Act, made the elimination of health care fraud the number one priority behind fighting violent crime, published numerous "guidances" for health care organizations, and dedicated billions of new dollars and hundreds of new agents to fighting fraud and abuse in health care. Predictably, the health care industry has responded to these government initiatives in ways that other industries have responded. It has established hundreds of new compliance programs and created thousands of new positions for compliance personnel. There is also evidence that other countries, particularly Australia, England, and Canada, are following the United States's lead in this area and are encouraging similar efforts of their own.

In response to these developments, the editors and authors of this volume believe that we could be witnessing the emergence or differentiation of a new profession. We discuss it here as the "compliance profession," and the practitioners in this new field as "compliance professionals." And, although we are not persuaded that the compliance profession is in fact a profession in the traditional sense of the term, we believe it could be good for society if such a profession were to take root and begin to mature.

Guide to Professional Development in Compliance begins to delimit, at least in broad strokes, this emerging profession and to address some of the needs around professional development for those who are now serving in it or hope to do so in the future. We also address a number of practical concerns that we hope will be of help to those working in compliance. Some of what our contributors write may be controversial, and some of what one contributor writes may contradict another. But we, as the editors, thought it important to begin the conversation in any case. In short, although we do not necessarily endorse every claim or argument made by our contributors, in this book we attempt to build on the momentum generated by the compliance movement in health care, both to address the concerns of compliance professionals generally and to bring the learning of compliance professionals in other industries and countries to bear on the problems facing professionals working in compliance. Thus, our focus here is on the compliance profession and the professional, in contrast to the compliance program. It is not so much a "how-to" book (although there is some of this), as it is a book that we hope will stimulate thinking and discussion about what it might mean for society generally should this occupation indeed emerge as a distinct profession and its practitioners undertake a sustained, rigorous, and self-critical program of professional development.

CHAPTER 1

Professional Ethical Development in Health Care Compliance

Mark E. Meaney

INTRODUCTION

Professional standards of conduct are born of individual and collective actions. They are not "learned at a mother's knee," but as part of a professional culture that professional associations develop through and sustain in community. Good qualities flourish with organizational support for ethical behavior. The opposite is a consequence of hostile circumstances. Professionals have a special relation to ethics because of the roles they occupy. More is appropriately expected of them because of their roles, not less.

This chapter addresses the subject of professional ethical development in health care compliance. Most people who work in the health care field consider themselves professionals. Some health care compliance professionals (HCCPs) even think of themselves as members of a distinct profession. The first part of this chapter argues that, in some respects, health care compliance ought to be considered a profession, albeit one in its formative stages. Moreover, HCCPs, individually and collectively, ought to be proactive in this regard: HCCPs should think and act as members of a distinct profession.

The second part of the chapter offers a program that would help the Health Care Compliance Association (HCCA) to further this goal. Because society entrusts a professional association with the regulation of the profession, such an association has a moral obligation to ensure that the members of the profession live up to professional standards of conduct. Professional ethical development is thus a moral obligation. It is the responsibility both of the professional association as a whole and of each of

1

its members. Although society has not yet officially recognized health care compliance as a profession through state licensure, HCCPs should be proactive in this regard, and accept this responsibility by continuing to develop as a profession, even if it is one that is in its early infancy.

What follows, then, is a blueprint for professional ethical development. This chapter presents guidelines for a program that could be implemented by HCCA in an effort to foster the development of professional ethical culture. If HCCA moves forward in this comprehensive undertaking, it should broaden the conversation to include as much input from as many quarters as possible. In fact, an important goal of such a program is to sustain a culture that encourages continued dialogue about fundamental value commitments. All HCCPs should take advantage of the opportunity to contribute to the legacy of the professional ethical development of the health care compliance profession.

"TO BE" OR "NOT TO BE" A PROFESSION

To properly address the professional status of HCCPs, terms must first be defined. What is a profession? This is a particularly pressing issue for HCCPs, as they seek clarity on their status in the health care industry. Is health care compliance a profession? Or, is it more akin to carpentry, plumbing, or auto mechanics, which are commonly referred to as *professional occupations*? Or, is it a subspecialty of another profession? If health care compliance is to become a profession, then it is important to remember that society affords the professions a great deal of autonomy. The professions are largely self-regulating and self-disciplinary. This level of professional autonomy thus comes with special moral or ethical responsibilities. Even though society has not yet recognized health care compliance as a profession (for example, by providing for state licensure), how can HCCA be proactive in this regard and fulfill moral obligations to cultivate professional ethical development? Finally, how ought HCCPs to comport themselves in a business environment?

To begin, it must be admitted that there is some controversy surrounding the definition of "profession." The way people commonly use the term reflects in language a certain degree of confusion.[1] In fact, some people who are called "professionals" are not members of a profession at all. Those in professional occupations do as full time work with a high degree of expertise what others do as a hobby, for pleasure, or in their spare time.

Various trades are considered professional occupations, for example, plumbers, carpenters, and mechanics. Further, some professional occupations do what many people do at an amateur level, for example, actors, athletes, and writers.

Conversely, members of a profession perform tasks that simply cannot be accomplished by the uninitiated. The word "profession" comes from the Latin word *professio*, which means a public declaration with the force of a promise. Members of a profession declare to the general public that they will act in certain ways, and that the group will discipline those who fail to do so. The profession presents itself to society as a social benefit; society, in turn, expects the profession to serve some important social goal.

The literature describes four essential characteristics that distinguish the professions:

1. competence in a specialized body of knowledge and skill
2. formalized education and accreditation
3. an acknowledgment of specific duties and responsibilities toward those they serve and toward society
4. the rights to train, admit, discipline, and dismiss its members for failure to sustain competence or observe special duties and responsibilities[2]

Medicine is often used as the paradigm example of a profession, with some justification. Physicians possess specialized skills and knowledge; they regulate access to that knowledge; they acknowledge special duties toward patients and society; and they discipline members for failure to observe their obligations as members of the profession. Finally, the state official recognizes the profession through state licensure.

Although the element of skill is an important characteristic, professional occupations often involve a higher degree of skill than many professions. For example, auto repair, cabinet making, and tool and die making involve more complex, intricate operations than school teaching, social work, or even nursing. The element of skill alone fails to distinguish the professions. The crucial distinction consists of a relation of skill to knowledge. A body of theoretical knowledge supports the skills of a member of a profession. Preparation for membership in a profession, therefore, involves formal education in an organized body of knowledge. Systematic theory is an essential prerequisite for practice in a profession.[3]

Members of a profession are also distinguished by the way that society accords them a greater degree of autonomy in the exercise of their authority than it does the trades, the arts, or business, because of the specialized nature of their skills and knowledge. Members of a profession establish their own standards and accreditation process, regulate entry into the field, and operate with relatively fewer social constraints. Such powers and privileges constitute a form of monopoly granted by society to members of a profession. In return for this singular degree of autonomy, members of a profession are expected to perform an important social function and serve the public good.[4]

The common distinction between "customers" and "clients" perhaps best illustrates how the professions perform an important social function. "Customers" have the capacity to know what they need and to judge whether a service or a commodity satisfies those needs. "Clients" lack the requisite knowledge to diagnose their needs and to judge the proper means to the proper ends. Although laypersons can judge certain aspects of the practice of members of a profession, clients are generally not competent to evaluate the quality of services rendered. Where a "customer" can criticize the quality of a commodity and perhaps demand a refund, clients must rely on experts to judge the competence of a member of a profession as well as to gain recourse in the event of malpractice.

The relation of client to a member of a profession is also more complex than customer to merchant. A businessperson is generally held to only the minimum moral standard of "do no harm" or "mitigate harm caused." Members of a profession, on the other hand, are held to a much higher standard than merely "do no harm." Members of a profession are expected to "pursue the good" of their clients.[5] Consequently, society expects professional associations to set higher standards of conduct for their members than those required of others, and to enforce a higher degree of discipline among their members than do professional occupations.

Is health care compliance a profession? It is doubtful whether a conclusive argument could be made one way or another in the space of a chapter, but the above characteristics can at least be used to make a preliminary determination. Does health care compliance differ in significant respects from professional occupations like auto mechanics or carpentry? It is clear that health care compliance entails a high degree of skill and knowledge. However, if health care compliance qualifies as a profession, then there must be a sufficient body of theoretical knowledge that would warrant a conclusion that systematic theory is a necessary prerequisite for practice. A cursory examination of the literature shows that development is underway of a body of knowledge that constitutes something like a systematic theory of health care compliance. One way to judge whether in fact there exists such a theory is to examine the literature to see whether alternate or competing theories are in place. Although it is perhaps too soon to tell, it seems probable that in the near future alternate interpretations of health care compliance theory will abound. In the meantime, the question remains open whether health care compliance meets this requirement. It is therefore an open question whether HCCPs are members of a profession on this basis.

The second criterion for membership in a profession is formal education and accreditation. Because of the specialized nature of health care compliance skill and knowledge, HCCA has begun to develop guidelines to regulate entry into the field by establishing an accreditation process and standards for the practice of health care compliance. Again, however, although HCCA has been proactive in this regard, in the absence of some form of state-enforced licensure, the question as to whether health care compliance will one day meet this requirement remains unanswered.

The third criterion of a profession is perhaps the most important. To qualify for the degree of professional autonomy normally reserved for members of a profession, society requires that the profession serve the public good. The earlier distinction between "customers" and "clients" can be used to illustrate how HCCPs perform a social function. Customers have the capacity to know what they need and to judge whether a service or a commodity satisfies those needs. HCCPs' clients, on the other hand, lack the requisite knowledge of health care compliance to diagnose their needs and to judge the proper means to the proper ends. Although clients may be able to judge certain aspects of the practice of health care compliance, they are not in the best position to evaluate the quality of services and must therefore trust HCCPs to complete the requisite tasks.

The third criterion also requires public acknowledgment of the specific duties and responsibilities that members of a profession have toward those they serve and toward society. Here again, HCCA has been proactive in helping HCCPs gain recognition as members of a profession. For example, the HCCA Code of Ethics for Health Care Compliance Professionals makes explicit the specific duties and responsibilities that all HCCPs have to the public. The first principle, "Obligations to the Public," states: "Health care compliance professionals should embrace the spirit and the letter of the law governing their professional affairs and exemplify the highest ethical standards in their conduct in order to contribute to the public good." HCCA thus acknowledges the special duties and responsibilities that HCCPs have toward society.

The fourth and last criterion of self-policing remains problematic for HCCPs and will remain so for the foreseeable future. A legally recognized profession has the right to discipline and dismiss members for failure to sustain competence or to observe their special duties and responsibilities. Absent state-enforced licensure, HCCA will find it difficult to enforce the Code through mechanisms of self-policing. Again, however, HCCA can be proactive here. This point is discussed in greater detail in the following sections.

It can be concluded, then, that health care compliance appears to satisfy some, but not all, of the four essential characteristics that mark a profession. Circumstances remain fluid. HCCPs possess a high degree of skill and specialized knowledge; they are in the process of establishing their own standards and accreditation process to regulate entry into the field; and they perform an essential service to the community. HCCA does not, however, have the state-enforced power to discipline members legally. The status of HCCPs as members of a profession, therefore, awaits the maturity of health care compliance as a practice in relation both to the law and to the health care system as a whole.

TOWARD PROFESSIONAL ETHICAL DEVELOPMENT IN HEALTH CARE COMPLIANCE

As suggested earlier, there is a trade-off between society and the professions. In exchange for more autonomy and less social control, the professions regulate and discipline members. In fact, society depends quite heavily upon the integrity of the professions. Although the state may sanction certification, only members of a profession are truly competent enough to determine the qualifications of members. Because society entrusts professional associations with the regulation of a profession, the profession has the moral obligation to ensure that members of a profession live up to professional standards of conduct. Professional ethical development is thus a moral obligation. It begins with the formation and dissemination of such a code of ethical conduct.[6]

If a code of ethical conduct is to serve as the basis upon which a profession can claim autonomy from social control, it must meet certain minimum requirements. A code should regulate the actual conduct of members of a profession and not merely list principles or unattainable ideals. It must provide evidence that the profession holds members accountable to the high moral standards expected by society of the profession members. In short, a code must demonstrate that the profession acts to protect the public interest as well as the interests of those it serves.

A code of ethical conduct should be specific and honest. It ought not merely state general moral guidelines, such as that members should not lie, cheat, or steal. Members of a profession know the potential pitfalls of a profession. They are in the best position to know how members might abuse information and power without public awareness of their activities. Only those with comparable knowledge can best restrain unprofessional or unethical conduct on the part of practitioners. A professional code should therefore specifically address those areas that pose as special temptations to members of a profession. It should regulate "shady" or questionable practices that, although not quite illegal, are nevertheless unethical.

Finally, a code ought to make provisions to bring accusations and to apply penalties in the case of illicit behavior. A code must be both policeable and policed. Society expects that a professional association will demonstrate that it can and does police its own ranks. If it should fail to do so, society has little reason to accord the profession special privileges, or a monopoly on information and power. When a profession proves incapable or even unwilling to police its own ranks, society is forced to legislate or micromanage activities, much as it does with other occupations.

As suggested earlier, HCCA has begun the hard work of professional ethical development with the dissemination of a code of ethics for HCCPs. The HCCA Code is discussed in greater depth in Chapter 5.[7] Suffice it here to say that the development of the Code was a truly monumental effort. The Code was submitted to every member of HCCA for comments. These members included government officials, attorneys, academics, consulting companies, and health care providers. The comments were numerous and overwhelmingly supportive; however, this is just a beginning.

Although a code of ethical conduct serves an important function, it can have several shortcomings. First, a code is not expository. Because it is not intended to be a text in moral theory, it does not of itself provide readers with an understanding of the derivation of moral principles. Readers are left to infer for themselves that the code's principles and moral rules have some basis other than mere consensus. For example, the HCCA Code of Ethics contains a Commentary. Although the Commentary expounds on the meaning of the rules, it does not provide readers with the theory that would be required ultimately to ground those rules, nor does it supply reasons as to why one should be moral in the first place. In short, a code is no substitute for an understanding of ethics and the foundations of professional ethics.

Second, a code gives little guidance on how to resolve morally ambiguous "hard cases" or new situations. For example, if HCCPs are to internalize the rules of their profession, they ought to be able to understand and apply moral principles to "hard cases" and new situations. The Code of Ethics cannot of itself provide HCCPs with the insight that is often necessary to resolve these complex, ethical conflicts. Thus, left standing alone, it is doubtful that a set of guidelines and rules will have a significant effect on behavior. A code of ethics becomes effective only when it is integrated into the culture of a profession and into the structures of a professional association.[8]

BUILDING PROFESSIONAL ETHICAL CULTURE

Every profession has its own distinctive ethos, culture, and value commitments. These unique characteristics derive from its own history and traditions, its own rules and ways of operating, and its own purposes and goals. Every profession also has its own particular place in a web of social and cultural relations. Members of a profession gain insight into professional ethical development, both as individuals and together as a community, by exploring the ethical values embedded in the culture and history of their own profession.

A professional association is founded at a particular time. Its original leaders import values, purposes, and goals into its charter. Their efforts give initial impetus and direction to the growth and development of the profession. Over time, the association and its subsequent leaders learn to respond to crises, to celebrate the good times, and to endure the bad. In this way, patterns of actions evolve both for the development of policy and for its implementation. These organizational patterns or habits entail specific value commitments. It is crucial to the health of a profession to make explicit the value commitments that are embedded within the original charter and policies of a professional association. The institutionalization of ethics across the profession depends on it, as does a profession's own unique identity. The articulation of and commitment to values are essential means by which a profession defines its own notions of professional integrity.[9]

Events and strong leaders mark the history of a profession. The past in this sense consists of a chronicle of the actions of a few for the sake of the many. Yet, the past is more that just what has happened. The sweat and toil of strong leaders lives on in the enduring values of the traditions or cultural heritage of a profession. Their work will continue to exert a powerful influence on the activity of the profession long after they have retired. Thus, history is not just what has happened in the past, but it is also what is remembered. The past is remembered not only through institutional structure and organizational habit, but it is also remembered through stories that are told about the lives and the practices of outstanding members of a profession. These stories are told over and over as part of the lore of a profession. They recount impossible barriers, difficult ethical dilemmas, and the moral courage of visionaries. The culture of every profession is a rich tapestry of vignettes, anecdotes, myths, and legends that convey shared values and beliefs. Professional ethical development involves tapping this rich vein of a profession's narrative to build commitment to its fundamental moral values throughout the membership.[10]

Thus, professional ethical development requires more than just a professional code of conduct, or a set of guidelines and rules. The institutionalization of value commitments across a profession requires: (1) the development of a professional ethical culture; (2) the integration of value commitments throughout the structures of the professional association; and (3) the fusion of ethical reflection into the daily practices of all members of the profession. Responsibility for professional ethical development must extend from national through regional leaders all the way to frontline practitioners in the field. This goal requires communication with and the involvement by all levels of the profession, and a commitment to professional ethical development. How to do this is one of the difficult problems that HCCA now faces.

For a profession to be infused with professional ethical culture means, first, that there are common understandings that unite members through a sense of community. Open communication is possible because there is an appreciation of a community of purpose. Second, professional ethical culture means that there is a strong sense of professional identity. Although members may perform diverse tasks, everyone feels like they are a part of the same profession and contribute in different ways to a shared mission. Third, professional ethical culture also entails a common understanding of professional integrity. Mere conformity to external guidelines or regulations does not yield professional integrity. Rather, solidarity based on common ethical values grounds professional integrity. As value commitments become explicit and institutionalized across the profession, habits of action reinforce cooperation and coordination beyond the legal minimum. Professional ethical culture takes root. Fourth, professional ethical culture means that there is a network of support that sustains participation and innovation. Members of a profession feel empowered to discuss sensitive or controversial ethical issues. Most important, they are confident in the knowledge that they have the support of a professional association in making the "hard choices" in the context of their own practice.[11]

In the development of professional ethical culture, it is important also to remember that a profession is a community. As a community, it consists of an organizational context of persons and groups, a system of customs, ethical values and purposes, and a network of actions and interactions. These are the essential building blocks for developing, shaping, and strengthening ethical culture within a profession. A professional association must: (1) tap the ethical resources of persons and groups; (2) develop the proper means to make explicit the fundamental values and principles of the profession; and (3) develop and sustain ethical leadership for the future.

A profession is, of course, made up of persons and groups in relation to the purposes of the profession. People bring their own natural talents, value commitments, and experiences with them into the setting of the professional community. Consequently, it is not necessary to start from scratch to develop and sustain professional ethical culture. The basic materials are already present among the people at work in the profession. A professional association should find a way to make use of this wealth of valuable experience. Of course, the individual ethics that people bring with them to a professional setting is not enough and needs shaping through professional ethical development. Nevertheless, in the development of professional ethical culture, it is a matter of incorporating the resources already present among members in order to remain in touch with evolving societal values.

As a community, a profession is also made up of a system of customs, values, and purposes. Customs evolve over time through relationships and actions that make up the social habits within a professional community. They may consist of various forms of ritual, ceremonies, conferences, celebrations, parties, and fun times that both represent the culture and serve to strengthen the infusion of values throughout the community. Customs, then, are an important vehicle for the development of professional ethical culture.

Values represent the goals and standards used by members of a profession for judging professional relations and actions as either better or worse. They provide criteria for evaluation. Over time, they shape and reshape the culture of a profession. The purposes of the profession express values in terms of goals for the future, and serve as the basis of change within the professional community. Together, customs, values, and purposes form the glue that binds a profession into a community. They come to be shared by members of a profession and form the basis of communication, and thus provide a network of commitments that inform action. It is therefore vital to the health of a professional community to make explicit its ethical values and goals so as to enhance communal relations. When members of a profession become more aware of the ethical foundations of their practice, they become more aware of themselves as part of a larger whole. As a consequence, they desire to learn and to apply principles to their work in an effort to further the legitimate interests of this greater whole.

Different professional associations have devised a variety of means to develop, sustain, and strengthen professional ethical culture. Some have chosen a more formal approach by relying on guidelines, rules, regulations, and procedures. Others have combined this formal approach with a more informal means of cultivating professional ethical culture. Although there are many examples of this latter tact, an important one can be found in the American Association of Engineering Societies and the National Society of Professional Engineers.[12] These professional associations have chosen to combine the adoption and dissemination of a code of ethics for engineers with the creation and publication of a more informal "ethics manual." Engineers recognize the shortcomings of codes of conduct and have chosen to supplement their code with a catalogue of "hard cases." The *Public Policy Perspectives and Positions*, together with the *Policy Statements and Papers*, amount to a narrative of the history of ethical reasoning in engineering.[13]

The associations draw upon the customs, the value commitments, and the experiences of the persons and groups within the profession in making explicit the fundamental ethical principles that ought to inform action. The ethics case studies contained in the manuals represent the lore of the profession of engineering, stories told over and over that recount seemingly impossible barriers, difficult ethical dilemmas, and the moral courage of visionaries. The culture of the profession is thus a mix of vignettes, anecdotes, myths, and legends that convey shared values and beliefs. Engineers have recognized that professional ethical development involves tapping this rich vein of the profession's narrative to build commitment throughout the profession to its fundamental moral values.

In their study of this more informal "ethics manual," members of the profession not only learn the principles and rules of ethical decision making contained in the code of engineering ethics, but they also learn how to apply those principles to "hard cases." The manual provides examples of concrete instances of how engineers in the past have resolved difficult moral dilemmas. Members of the profession thereby gain insight into the professional ethical culture of engineering. They come to appreciate the common understandings of ethical values that unite engineers in a professional community. Consequently, members of the profession develop a strong sense of professional identity and integrity. As value commitments have become explicit and institutionalized across the profession, habits of action have reinforced cooperation and coordination among engineers beyond a legal or formal framework. Professional engineering associations have developed a network of support that sustains participation and innovation. Ethical culture empowers members of the profession to discuss sensitive or controversial ethical issues. Most important, the culture creates confidence in the knowledge that members have the support of a professional association in making the "hard choices" in the context of their own engineering practice.

Moreover, professional engineering societies have taken a number of steps to ensure the translation of ethical culture into the structures and institutions of professional associations. The professional code of conduct and informal "ethics manuals" provide a framework for regional and national advisory councils, ethics committees, and commissions. Such professional boards not only serve as a venue for the review of breaches in the professional code of conduct or ethical culture, but they also function as a mechanism for the promotion of ethical reflection throughout all levels of the profession. Ethics committees and commissions sponsor conferences and professional bulletins that keep members of the profession abreast of changes in societal values, engineering ethics, and related legal issues. To get as much input from as many quarters as possible, the American Association of Engineering Societies promotes through its publications and programs multidisciplinary group discussions on professional ethics.

Ethics training is fast becoming mandatory for all engineering students in universities and colleges across the country. The purpose of this initiative is to introduce students both to the professional ethical culture of engineering and to the structures and institutions that support it. The added benefit, of course, is that the profession creates a pool of ethical leadership for the future. Institutional leadership is essential for the promotion and protection of professional values. Ethics training ensures that the values and purposes of the profession remain at the core of a professional ethical culture that sustains and enhances public trust.

IMPLICATIONS FOR HEALTH CARE COMPLIANCE

The task, then, that lies before HCCA may be interpreted as follows. In general terms, absent state licensure, HCCA should continue to be proactive and fulfill special moral obligations to society consequent upon the status of a professional association. These special moral obligations would constitute a kind of implied contract between society and HCCA in lieu of official state recognition. Because society entrusts professional associations with the regulation of the profession, HCCA should continue to accept professional ethical development as a moral obligation. It would, therefore, be a responsibility both of the professional association as a whole and of each of its members.

As discussed, professional ethical development begins with the formation and dissemination of a professional code of conduct. Such a code must indicate that the members of a profession intend to act to protect the public interest as well as the interests of those they serve. HCCA has already begun work on professional ethical development with the adoption and dissemination of a code of conduct, but this is just a beginning. Although codes serve an important function, it has been noted that they fail to provide members of a profession with insight into both the ground of moral principles generally and the justification of the moral life. Although the Commentary of the Code of Ethics begins the process, readers should seek the help of trained ethicists to understand its basis fully. In addition, codes give little guidance on how to resolve morally ambiguous "hard cases" or new situations. If HCCPs are to internalize the rules of their profession, they must understand how those rules are derived, and how to apply moral principles to "hard cases" and new situations. Left standing alone, it is doubtful that the HCCA's Code of Ethics for Health Care Compliance Professionals will have a significant effect on behavior. In fact, it can be argued that such a code will become effective only when it is integrated into the culture of a profession and into the structures of a professional association.

In more specific terms, then, professional ethical development for health care compliance requires more than just a professional code of conduct, or a set of guidelines and rules. As suggested earlier, the institutionalization of value commitments generally, and in health care compliance specifically, requires: (1) the development of a professional ethical culture; (2) the integration of value commitments throughout the structures of HCCA; and (3) the fusion of ethical reflection into the daily practices of all HCCPs. Responsibility for professional ethical development in health care compliance must extend from HCCA national leaders through HCCA regional leaders to HCCPs in the field. Again, this goal requires communication with, involvement of, and commitment to professional ethical development at all levels of health care compliance.

From what was said earlier, it can be concluded that to achieve this goal, HCCA must continue to: (1) tap the ethical resources of persons and groups in health care compliance; (2) develop the means to make explicit the fundamental values and principles of health care compliance; and (3) develop and sustain ethical leadership for the future of the profession. Professional associations have chosen a variety of means to develop, sustain, and strengthen professional ethical culture. Some have chosen a more formal approach by relying strictly on codes, guidelines, rules, and regulations. Others have combined this formal approach with a more informal means of cultivating professional ethical culture. Health care compliance would do well to adopt this latter approach.

In adopting this approach, HCCA should follow the lead of other professional associations by drawing upon the customs, the value commitments, and the experiences of the persons and groups within health care compliance to make explicit the fundamental ethical principles that ought to inform action. The young culture of health care compliance has already given rise to vignettes and anecdotes that convey shared values and beliefs. Engineers have recognized that professional ethical development involves tapping this vein of a profession's narrative to build commitment to its fundamental moral values throughout the profession. HCCPs ought to do the same. HCCPs have a unique opportunity in this regard, as they stand at the very beginnings of the emergence of their profession. This is a distinct advantage. The original visionaries and leaders of health care compliance yet live and practice. This provides a unique opportunity to gather together the stories that comprise the original narrative of health care compliance. The vignettes and anecdotes of the "first ones" of any profession tell a narrative about the fundamental values and principles that ought to inform practice. One need only tap this reservoir.

A three-step process will complete this task. First, an ethics survey could canvas the opinions of a cross-section of HCCPs. The survey would accomplish two things: (1) it would provide an indication of the extent to which HCCPs have an appreciation for the importance of professional ethical development and culture, and (2) it would help to determine whether HCCPs, individually and collectively, take seriously their implied contract with society. Also, the survey would provide data for progress toward professional ethical culture. It would inquire about specific events and cases. The questions would be tailored to help HCCPs reflect on the ethical content of "hard cases."

Second, once the data are collected and analyzed, the ideas and ethical reflections of this cross-section could be used to compile a sampling of the most difficult ethical dilemmas in health care compliance. Then a list of specific questions could be formulated and these ethical dilemmas could be worked up into sample cases. The questions and cases could be categorized according to specific topics that pose particular difficulties. Then these questions and cases could be used in a series of interviews with some of the original leaders and visionaries of health care compliance. Both their answers to the questions and their responses to "hard cases" could then be recorded on videotape. The material would then be edited to produce a series of educational videos for the benefit of national and regional leaders as well as for HCCPs in the field.

The video series could be used to capture the lore of the profession of health care compliance, those stories that will be told over and over again about impossible odds, ethical conflicts, and the moral courage of the original visionaries. The series could help to strengthen and sustain the professional ethical culture of health care compliance, so that both new and old members could appreciate the common ethical values that hold HCCPs together in a professional community.

In the third step of this process, the materials from the ethics survey and from the interviews could be gathered together to produce ethics literature for health care compliance by way of an "ethics manual." As in engineering, an ethics manual for health care compliance would supplement the professional code of conduct. The manual would provide a means by which HCCPs can both learn the principles and rules of ethical decision making contained in the code of conduct and how to apply those principles to "hard cases." Just as in engineering, the manual would provide examples of concrete instances of how professionals in the past have resolved difficult moral dilemmas. HCCPs would thereby gain insight into not only the code of conduct, but also the professional ethical culture of health care compliance.

Recall that for a profession to be infused with professional ethical culture means, first, that there are common understandings that unite members through a sense of community. Open communication about difficult issues is possible because there is an appreciation of a community of purpose. Second, it means that there is a strong sense of professional identity. Everyone feels like part of the same profession and contributes in different ways to a shared mission. To further this end, the results of the three-step process described earlier could be used to provide a framework for ethics training across the profession. The training would begin at the national and regional levels and would take the form of a series of conferences to disseminate pertinent materials.[14] The conferences could be designed as forums to advance discussion on important ethical and legal issues and as a means to "train the trainers."

As value commitments become explicit and institutionalized across the profession, habits of action will reinforce continued cooperation and coordination among HCCPs beyond a mere formal framework. HCCA would, in effect, develop a network of support that sustains participation and innovation. Ethical culture will empower HCCPs to discuss sensitive or controversial ethical issues. Most important, the culture would create confidence in the knowledge that members have the support of HCCA in making the "hard choices" in the context of their own practices.

HCCA can take a number of steps to build organizational support in order to ensure that professional ethical culture gets translated into the structures and institutions of the association. The professional code of conduct and informal ethics manuals for health care compliance can provide a framework for regional and national advisory councils, ethics committees, and commissions. As in engineering, such professional boards will not only serve as a venue for the review of breaches in the professional code of conduct or ethical culture, but they can also function as a mechanism for the promotion of ethical reflection throughout all levels of the profession.

Health care compliance advisory boards and ethics committees can sponsor conferences and professional bulletins that keep members of the profession abreast of changes in societal values, professional ethics, and related legal issues. Finally, HCCA can promote through its publications and programs multidisciplinary group discussions on professional ethics to get as much input from as many members as possible.

CONCLUSION

This chapter has suggested that professional ethical development is a moral obligation both of HCCA and of each of its members. It has also suggested that there is a strong practical benefit, as it would further the long-term goal of official recognition of health care compliance as a profession. A blueprint for professional ethical development must foster the development of professional ethical culture. An important goal is to develop and to sustain a culture that encourages continued dialogue about the fundamental value commitments of health care compliance. If HCCA moves forward in such a comprehensive undertaking, the conversation ought to include as much input from as many quarters as possible. It is this author's hope that everyone in the field would take advantage of a unique opportunity to contribute to the legacy of the profession ethical development of health care compliance.

NOTES

1. M.S. LARSON, THE RISE OF PROFESSIONALISM: A SOCIOLOGICAL ANALYSIS (1977).

2. E. FREIDSON, PROFESSIONAL DOMINANCE (1970).

3. R.H. Hall, *Professionalism and Bureaucratization*, 33 AM. Soc. REV. 92–104 (1968).

4. A.H. GOLDMAN, THE MORAL FOUNDATIONS OF PROFESSIONAL ETHICS (1980).

5. M.D. BAYLES, PROFESSIONAL ETHICS (2d ed. 1989).

6. P.Y. WINDT ET AL., ETHICAL ISSUES IN THE PROFESSIONS (1989).

7. *See* Chapter 5, *Thinking Like a Compliance Professional: The HCCA Code of Ethics for Health Care Compliance Professionals.*

8. E.D. TERRENCE & A.A. KENNEDY, CORPORATE CULTURES: THE RITES AND RITUALS OF CORPORATE LIFE (1982).

9. J.R. Phillips & A.A. Kennedy, *Shaping and Managing Shared Values*, 12 MCKINSEY STAFF PAPER 4 (1980).

10. M. Goldberg, *Corporate Culture and the Corporate Culture, in* A VIRTUOUS LIFE IN BUSINESS 29–50 (O.F. Williams & J.W. Houck eds., 1992).

11. J.R. Phillips & A.A. Kennedy, *Shaping and Managing Shared Values*, 12 MCKINSEY STAFF PAPER 5 (1980).

12. M.W. MARTIN & R. SCHINZINGER, ETHICS IN ENGINEERING (1983).

13. R.A. GORLIN, CODES OF PROFESSIONAL RESPONSIBILITY (1990).

14. To its credit, HCCA has included an ethics course as part of its Academy for Health Care Compliance. Of course, what is described here goes well beyond a single course offering.

CHAPTER 2

The Compliance Officer: Delimiting the Domain

Joseph E. Murphy

INTRODUCTION

When a new position is introduced into the corporate world, one of the first challenges is to determine how this new role differs from existing roles. What is the job of the person who occupies this new position? Should others in the organization see the new person as a threat or an ally? How do others know when the person has overstepped his or her bounds?

The compliance officer and other compliance positions are relatively new to the health care industry. Following the dramatic increase in investigations and government enforcement actions in health care, compliance offices have sprung up at an unprecedented rate. In this environment of rapid development and deployment, it is important to step back and examine the limits of the compliance domain.

The development of formal compliance programs has been driven by government initiatives, so the first point of reference is the standards set by government. Chapter 8 of the 1991 United States Sentencing Guidelines[1] sets the standards for the minimum elements needed for an effective compliance program. These influential standards include this statement:

> Specific individual[s] within high-level personnel of the organization must have been assigned overall responsibility to oversee compliance with [the organization's compliance] standards and procedures.[2]

"High-level personnel" is defined to mean those with substantial control over the organization or who have a substantial role in making policy.[3]

Examples include directors, executive officers, those in charge of major business or functional units, and individuals with substantial ownership interest.

Although the compliance oversight position has been referred to by different names, including ethics officer, compliance officer, and combinations of those two, this chapter uses "compliance officer" for convenience of reference. For the most part this chapter discusses the role of the compliance professional from the perspective of the highest level—that of compliance officer. But there are a number of subordinate positions that make a compliance program work. These can include assistant compliance officers, compliance committee members, attorneys who are assigned to the program, and members of other departments who work regularly with the compliance office such as internal audit, security, human resources, corporate communications, environmental affairs, and safety. It also includes subsidiary and business unit compliance representatives. The points made in this chapter about the compliance officer's domain should also guide the role of these other "players."

THE COMPLIANCE OFFICER'S ROLE DEFINED

The nature of the compliance officer's responsibilities is essentially defined by the Sentencing Guidelines list of items expected to be included in the compliance program. It is clear from looking at this list of functions that the chief compliance officer has substantial administrative and managerial responsibility. This person is charged with responsibility for implementing a companywide program with an ambitious agenda—to prevent and detect wrongdoing.

Following the lead of the Sentencing Guidelines, the Office of Inspector General (OIG) of the Department of Health and Human Services (HHS) issued guidelines on compliance programs for various participants in the health care industry.[4] These guidelines, or guidance documents, offer more detail on the compliance officer and an additional infrastructure item, the compliance committee. From the OIG's perspective, the compliance officer is the "focal point for compliance activities." The key functions of the compliance officer, according to this document, are "coordination and communication." The OIG then provides a list of functions that belong to the compliance program, basically elaborating on the list in the Sentencing Guidelines.

The OIG also recommends creation of a compliance committee to advise and assist the compliance officer in implementing the program. The listed functions of this committee then track the various elements of the compliance program, such as assessing policies and procedures and developing a system to solicit, evaluate, and respond to complaints and problems.

In the legal environment, one would usually look to cases to elaborate on such standards as set by the Guidelines and the OIG guidance documents. But it is the nature of serious lawbreaking allegations against major business entities in the United States that they do not go to trial, but rather end in settlements. Thus, there have not been helpful litigated cases thus far. What cases have appeared have been in the civil context. In the Caremark Derivative litigation, the Delaware Chancery court indicated that board members of corporations could face personal liability for ignoring the value of a compliance information system.[5] In cases in the employment discrimination area, including sexual harassment, courts, starting with the U.S. Supreme Court, have opined that compliance programs can act as a defense, either to liability[6] or to punitive damages.[7] In none of these cases has there been much attention to the role of compliance professionals, but the potential remains for further guidance from the judiciary. One strong message is emerging from these cases, however; namely, that robust compliance programs have an important role to play in protecting companies, not just in the criminal environment, but in civil litigation as well. At a minimum, this instructs that the domain of the compliance professional cannot be limited to the criminal law, but must extend to other areas where the company faces exposure for wrongdoing. It also means that the compliance professional needs the authority to ensure that the compliance program is an effective one, and not simply a paper sham.

The law, in effect, asserts that the scope of the compliance professional's job is potentially as broad as the range of legal liability, and that this person must be an able manager who can ensure that the company embraces a robust program. None of this legal guidance, however, dictates a detailed borderline between the compliance officer and other actors in the corporate environment.

Thus, beyond the legal parameters, a second question to ask about the compliance officer is whether this person is the conscience of the company. Many years ago the author heard of a general counsel who pointedly announced that his law department was not the conscience of the corporation. This was a general counsel who was noted for not welcoming challenges to his views, and who obviously did not want his staff diverted from what he viewed as the traditional legal department role. Attorneys give advice; the managers decide what to do with that advice.

This remark highlights two separate questions. The first is whether there is a need for any conscience function in corporations. If the answer to that is, "Yes," then the next question is, "Who?" What officer or department should serve as the corporation's conscience?

The message from the government is that there is a need for more than someone who merely opines on the rules, but then bears no responsibility for what happens next. This level of passivity now stands as a hallmark of the company that is not a good citizen corporation. To meet the new standard, companies must have a system and an organization in place to affirmatively interdict wrongdoing. Thus, the answer seems to be that there must be a voice in the organization that not only objects to wrongdoing, but also one with the ability to prevent and detect misconduct.

Yet it cannot be accurate to say that a compliance officer and a small cadre of in-house compliance professionals are the only ones responsible for ensuring that the company does the right thing. As the HCCA Code of Ethics for Health Care Compliance Professionals specifically spells out: "While [compliance professionals] should exercise a leadership role in compliance assurance, all employees have the responsibility to ensure compliance."[8] Thus, although the compliance officer may set the systems in place to ensure that management considers the right thing to do, it will always be up to all the employees to give life to the company's compliance commitment.

The question about a corporate conscience leads into another difficult question. What is the standard of performance that is being addressed by the compliance officer? When the Sentencing Guidelines were initially promulgated, some attorneys literally looked at the scope of the specific criminal laws covered by the Guidelines, and took that to be the limit of the compliance domain. In one major company, for example, the chief attorney proudly announced at a conference that a staff member had reviewed all of Title 18 of the United States Code, the title dealing with federal crimes, to see what the company's compliance program should cover.

In fact, however, companies soon realized that no matter how much legal training is provided, employees do not see the compliance world as confined to Title 18. If a system is established to deal with wrongdoing, employees will use it to address what they view as improper conduct. If the company arbitrarily cuts off such inquiry, it will severely limit the appeal and understanding of the company's compliance reporting system. The best practice among compliance programs has moved to covering a broader notion of wrongdoing. Whether it is denominated ethics, values, "doing the right thing," or integrity, it is no longer expected that employees will parse the statute books to determine the scope of the program. Companies now address a broad range of wrongdoing and misconduct, and press their employees to act not just within the law, but ethically as well. This is reflected in the fact that the largest cross-industry organization of compliance professionals, the Ethics Officer Association,[9] does not even use the term "compliance" in the name of the organization, even though compliance is probably the most common *raison d'être* for its members.

This shift to a broader "values" focus is not just a response to employee perception. It is also a recognition that the standards set in the Sentencing Guidelines could be read to require such an approach, if this is what makes the program effective.[10] The Guidelines were written to be flexible[11]; they require diligence, effectiveness, and a system at least as good as industry practice. If others in the same industry conclude that a values focus is necessary to make the program effective, this may become the applicable legal standard for effectiveness. Thus, even if management intends the program only to prevent and detect criminal wrongdoing, it may nevertheless be necessary to include a values orientation as the only way to make the program actually work and meet the standards of the Guidelines.

If it is accepted that a modern compliance program must reach beyond mere minimum legal standards, and that no one individual or unit in a corporation can function exclusively as the conscience of the organization, then where does that put the compliance officer and the other compliance professionals? The answer is that the compliance officer is the manager responsible for creating the processes that will increase the likelihood that the company will do the right thing. The compliance officer need not make the decisions about what is right and wrong, but that officer seeks to ensure that decisions made by the company seriously take that question into consideration.

Thus, the compliance officer and the compliance organization strive to inform employees about the rules that apply. They devise systems so that questions about right and wrong rise to the top, such as hotlines and regular reporting systems that reach the senior executives and the board of directors. They examine the incentive systems in the organization so that those systems lead employees to do the right thing. And they ensure that there are systems to check on the employees' performance to see that they are, in fact, doing what is right.

The compliance officer is the manager of the compliance and ethics process. In this respect this officer is comparable to an organization's chief financial officer (CFO).[12] For a business to be successful, all employees have to have bottom-line accountability and be responsible for revenue and expense. But there is still one officer responsible for managing the system and ensuring that controls are in place.

Similarly, the compliance officer sees to it that all necessary parts of the compliance program are in place and working. This officer oversees the infrastructure, including the business unit compliance programs, the management of the various compliance risk areas, and the specific elements as detailed in the Sentencing Guidelines, in the OIG Guidances, and in the standards of other agencies.[13]

To further refine this view of the compliance officer, it is also useful to look at what the compliance officer is not. As noted earlier, the compliance officer cannot be the repository of all compliance responsibility; all employees must share that responsibility. But there is another critical role that the compliance officer cannot fulfill alone. One of the anomalies of the Sentencing Guidelines is that they do not explicitly contain the most commonly offered advice on compliance programs: that no program can truly succeed without the support of senior management. Books, articles, speeches—whether on compliance, ethics, or anything related to this subject—almost always make this point, usually as the first requirement for success. Yet the Guidelines do not.

The Guidelines' reference to a high-level person in charge is taken as a surrogate for this point. But in literally following the Guidelines it is possible to overlook the importance of the support of senior executives. It is true that an empowered and skilled compliance officer can make a great difference in the effectiveness of a compliance program, and such an officer may have excellent access to other senior officers. But this is not necessarily the same as active senior officer support.

Senior executives still must set the tone at the top of an organization. Employees throughout the organization will look to see what really matters to the people at the top of the pyramid. If those officers live the values of the program, if they speak out in its support and actually are guided by it in their own conduct, this will contribute mightily to the program's impact. In this context, it is thus not the job of the compliance officer to play the roles of the chief executive and the rest of the senior officers. The compliance officer's role is not to be their ethical stand-in. Rather, the value the compliance officer brings is as a champion of the program among the senior managers. The compliance officer provides guidance to them, but they in turn lead the business and determine the real commitment to ethical conduct.

There is also a legal dimension to this emphasis on the separate role of the senior executives. Legally, the organization will be liable if the officers are involved in wrongdoing, no matter how good the program and the compliance officer may be. The government is not likely to accept an argument based on a "rogue executives" theory. No matter how honest and law-abiding the great mass of employees may be, and no matter how diligently the compliance officer may perform, if the senior executives are engaged in or condone illegal conduct, the organization will face tough enforcement and full liability at the hands of the legal system.

Another boundary for the compliance function is that it does not perform the policing of business-oriented rules or the management of business functions. For example, compliance would not include such business performance measurements as assessing who meets the targeted sales objectives for each business unit. Similarly, compliance is not the enforcement of attendance rules, or the performance of standard human resources administrative functions. What is the distinction that is intended here? The standards addressed by the compliance program are ones that are, for the most part, externally imposed and enforced. They are primarily to protect others in society from the power of the organization. They are not the types of standards, like sales quotas, that can be readily adjusted to meet business needs.

This distinction is not an absolute one, and it is common for compliance programs to contain elements designed to protect the company from being the target of wrongdoing. But even in that environment, the focus is based on law and ethics, not business performance standards. For example, conflicts of interest standards help protect the company from having its employees' loyalties diverted by vendors' gifts and other favors. Yet there are ethical and legal dimensions to this as well. Lavish gifts and favors can cross the line under legal standards for commercial bribery, antikickback statute violations, tax evasion, conspiracy, and other actionable violations. Similarly, protection of company proprietary information as a compliance function can overlap with legal restrictions on insider trading, and is often connected with the compliance issue of protecting and respecting others' confidential information. By contrast, business management is much further removed from these types of externally imposed standards.

COMPARISON TO OTHER PROFESSIONS AND MANAGEMENT POSITIONS

The previous discussion gives the basic picture of how the compliance officer's role is defined. To give this more context, it is useful to compare the compliance role to existing functions in organizations that may perform similar tasks.

The General Counsel and the Legal Department

Perhaps the most obvious comparison of the compliance officer's role is to the corporate legal department. When the Sentencing Guidelines were first promulgated, it was common for companies almost automatically to designate the general counsel, or another attorney, as the compliance officer. After all, the logic went, compliance was a legal matter, and who better to tackle this task than an attorney. Over time, however, many companies realized that compliance was more about management than law, and that although the compliance officer needed a good attorney, that officer did not need to *be* an attorney.

How do the two roles differ? The attorney's orientation is centrally focused on protecting the client, conditioned by the combat environment of litigation. The attorney is ethically obligated to be "zealous" in the client's defense. This standard may tend to make counsel somewhat less inclined to embrace the policing model in dealing with the corporate client. Indeed, attorneys are often advised to be constructive in dealing with the clients, and to suggest ways for the client to achieve its objectives within the law. There is certainly nothing wrong with this advice, and it does facilitate the legal counseling role. This advice reflects a basic point about dealing with others. One can be a counselor or one can be a cop, but it is difficult to play the same role with the same people. If corporate counsel is viewed as the internal police, there is likely to be much less willingness on the part of managers to approach counsel for advice.

The compliance officer, too, needs to play a consultative role.[14] But this position must engage in auditing, monitoring, and investigations as well. This gives the function a sharper edge, much closer to that of auditors.

Legal counsel may also be less inclined to engage in postmortems after a problem is uncovered. Rather, counsel is often required to move on quickly to fight the next fire; there is rarely time to sift through the ashes of the last fire to determine the cause. The compliance officer, in contrast, is obligated to devote attention to the determination of the causes of past failures. The message of item 7 of the Guidelines standards makes this clear.[15]

Legal counsel also is conditioned to be especially alert for the need to protect client confidential communication. The ability to protect privilege is enhanced when the number of participants in any communication is limited. The practice of law is not a consumer-oriented, mass retail type of operation. The historic model, rather, is of the individual attorney consulting in confidence with the individual client.

The compliance role shares some of this need for confidence and privilege. In the current environment, where the legal system has been spotty in recognizing the need to protect compliance-related activities from exploitation in litigation, the usual course is to bring in counsel at sensitive points to protect communications. Thus, for investigations, it is often necessary to turn matters over to counsel. However, the compliance officer has a mass-education and control function as well. Unlike the attorney, the compliance officer is a creature of mass organizations. The position does not function at an optimum level shrouded in secrecy. The officer does not just give advice to managers who then must implement it. Instead, the officer must determine how to train, assess, and monitor every employee of the company in the legal and ethical standards that apply. The model is not the individual counseling one; it is, instead, closer to the mass advertising field.

One critical distinction between the compliance officer and attorneys in the legal department is that the compliance officer does not perform legal analysis, manage litigation, or provide legal advice. Rather, the compliance officer goes to legal counsel to obtain such advice and assistance. The compliance officer may then take the advice of counsel and apply it in performing his or her compliance management functions.

Most of these observations, except for the limits on actual legal practice, are not intended as absolutes, but merely as differences in orientation. One point where counsel and the compliance officer are well aligned, however, is the need to approach the function from an outsider's perspective. Every compliance program exists to perform at least two functions. The first is an internal function—to affect employees' behavior. The second is an external function—to be able to convince an outsider that the company was serious about compliance and was a good citizen corporation. To meet this latter test the compliance officer needs to maintain an external orientation. There must always be an eye on how things would look to a skeptical prosecutor, regulator, or newspaper reporter. Like the attorney, the compliance officer must always have in mind the worst case, and must have the ability to look at corporate activities from a skeptical outsider's perspective.

Internal Audit

A second useful point of comparison is the internal audit department and the auditing profession. For internal audit, more than for the legal profession, internal policing is a focus. True auditing is not managing or counseling; it is, instead, a core part of the control system that management installs to ensure that its directions and standards are followed. In this context, enlightened auditors may provide advice on how to fix problems that are found, but in the first instance the role is one of controlling conduct.

Internal audit has also provided one of the most important models for empowering corporate compliance organizations—the relationship to the board of directors. At least in the top tier of publicly traded companies, the internal audit organization has a direct reporting relationship to the audit committee, composed of nonmanagement directors. The chief auditor can meet with these board members in executive session, and is obligated to report anomalies or problems posed by management that might interfere with the auditors' control functions. Companies have adopted this model to similarly empower their compliance operations.

Internal audit, like the compliance function, is accustomed to unobstructed access to facilities, files, and personnel in the organization. Again, this same model has guided the compliance officer, and is part of the HCCA Code of Ethics for Health Care Compliance Professionals.[16]

One trait that attorneys and auditors share is the existence of professional standards. This helps insulate each group from the pressures of company management. No matter what direction may come from the senior managers of an organization, a professional cannot afford to violate these professional standards; doing so can cause the person to lose the ability to practice his or her profession—a cost too high for the professional. As a result of the HCCA's groundbreaking efforts, health care compliance professionals are now moving into the professional category, with their own set of ethical standards.

Compliance officers are distinguished from auditors, however, by their counseling and managing roles. They cannot simply be police on the beat. They must also implement the broad-ranging management elements of a compliance program. They must be available to consult on ethical and code of conduct issues, which requires the balance described in Chapter 3.[17]

The Finance Control System and the Chief Financial Officer

Related to the audit function are the larger finance organization and the CFO. The financial organization typically has a control orientation, including as it does the internal audit organization. But the prevailing orientation is numbers and money. Compliance, by contrast, covers a broader range of human conduct. Some of the compliance function is financially related, such as compliance with books and records standards. But other risk areas, such as sexual harassment, deal with human conduct at its most basic level, with no specific relationship to finances.

The financial organization and the CFO are also closer to being part of the normal management team. Unlike auditing and compliance, they are focused on the bottom line, and play a more participatory role in development of the business.

Risk Management

Compliance is not the only function that is focused on assessing and controlling risks. The risk assessment organization also has a control orientation. This group recognizes the need to identify and address risks faced by the business. This is certainly an element shared with compliance, but with some key differences.

Risk management assesses risks in a context where the target is to reduce the risks to an acceptable level. There is recognition that risks, like fire, theft, and sharp changes in the economy, are considered inevitable, but that there are steps that can reduce or ameliorate these risks. In the compliance arena it may well be true that all risk of wrongdoing cannot be eliminated. But the notion of "acceptable risks" when connected with serious wrongdoing is simply not acceptable to society, and can be deadly when paraded in front of a jury. It is acceptable to calculate the risks of a flood and then take cost-justified steps to address that risk. It is not acceptable to perform the same calculations regarding deaths from product poisoning, or to do a cost–benefit analysis that includes the projected impact of a criminal fine for bribery.

Risk management is also more business oriented than compliance. After risk management identifies a risk, it is a matter of business judgment whether and how to ameliorate the risk. This environment does not deal with the impact of whistleblowers, *qui tam* suits, grand jury investigations, or angry citizens. In the compliance context, legal standards play a much larger role, limiting the business freedom. Under *Caremark*,[18] boards have a duty to have a system to monitor compliance; it is not just a business management decision. Being aware of a problem and failing to act can lead to potential liability for the organization, and loss of the benefit that would otherwise derive from having a diligent compliance program.

Risk management is typically in an advisory or consultative role. It is not typically associated with strong policing and management duties. By contrast, the compliance office has a duty to take a more active role, driving the entity to do the right thing.

Human Resources

Another active "player" in areas dealing with compliance is the human resources (HR) department. The typical HR portfolio contains important compliance functions, including employment discrimination and the related issue of harassment, compliance with immigration requirements (that is, I-9 forms), and protection of employee privacy. HR people are often familiar, even highly experienced, with the legal landscape.

Another advantage HR staff brings to the compliance environment is that they tend to be process oriented. HR includes processes that are critical in giving real impact to a compliance program. HR staff will typically address the hiring and termination processes, as well as assessments and discipline. These are core parts of compliance with which other groups, including legal and even internal audit, may not be as familiar.

HR differs from compliance in part because it is often not as oriented or comfortable with the types of legal, hard-core misconduct such as bribery, health care fraud, and price-fixing, which must be a major focus of compliance. They also lack the strength of an established professional standard, and are subject to greater pressure to go along with the rest of management. They tend to be more aligned with the consulting side, with some strength in policing in their specialty areas. Their management role extends to the

HR functions. This management function includes the more mundane administrative roles, such as getting payroll details in order. In all of these roles HR tends organizationally to have less clout than is appropriate for an effective compliance program.

Corporate Security

The in-house security organization, where it exists, may play a strong compliance-related role, or it may be only a marginal operation, depending on the nature of the business. In retail, for example, security might be nothing more than store guards who watch out for shoplifters. In high-tech fields, prevention of the theft or misuse of proprietary information or invasion of high-tech fortresses may lead companies to have a sophisticated security function, skilled in investigations of a broader range of wrongdoing. In this latter category, security can bring valuable skills to the compliance program. But even the best security organization will be limited to the role of policing.

Quality Control

Quality control is typically oriented toward ensuring that the company produces safe and reliable products, or provides services at a certain level of competency. Quality control shares with compliance a focus on process. Effective quality and effective compliance require certain controls and processes to minimize the opportunity for errors. Compliance and quality control also share a mission of determining the root causes of troubles when they occur. This includes scrutiny of all elements of a process, not just the specific point where the last step of a violation occurred.

Quality control does not, however, usually deal with willful offenders, which is a characteristic of compliance. Those who make innocent production mistakes may need only to be retrained or given better guides for their daily business activities. Willful offenders, however, are not in need of more training. Rather, they need a harsher edge to the program, including audits, investigations, and discipline strong enough to act as a deterrent.

The Ombuds Position

Some companies have a designated neutral—an ombuds—whom employees can call with a variety of concerns and issues. For the pure ombuds, the chief function is that of advisor and mediator. The ombuds does not investigate, recommend discipline, or suggest new organizational structures to address wrongdoing. Rather, this office provides an ear for the concerned or disgruntled employee.

This ombuds role does serve important compliance purposes. When presented with information about wrongdoing, the ombuds can advise the employee to contact the compliance office. The ombuds is also supposed to be truly independent, not reporting to company management or taking management's side in disputes. This emphasis on independence resembles one of the elements of a compliance position, and serves to surface issues that might otherwise remain buried.

The ombuds role has some distinct differences from compliance, however. Most important, an ombuds risks being marginalized or viewed as a gadfly. Other than the power of persuasion, it does not appear that the ombuds has the "clout" or the power to make things happen in the organization. There is no management or policing role, only consulting. The compliance officer must be a "player"; the ombuds stands alone.

Inspectors General

One last organizational unit worth considering is the office of inspector general, usually found in government agencies. There have been circumstances where private versions of such offices, called independent private sector inspectors general (IPSIG) have been instituted in companies.[19] These offices tend to function exclusively on the policing model. They are there to detect wrongdoing, and thus act as a deterrent to misconduct. In the government setting they are made independent of those they are asked to police. They do not have the consulting or management roles that characterize the compliance office, and can thus operate with the greater hostility likely to characterize relations with a policing group.

DEFINING THE POSITION: THE HCCA'S ETHICAL STANDARDS

A look at the boundaries of the compliance professional would be incomplete without taking into account the HCCA ethical standards.[20] These are especially enlightening because they spell out the three levels of responsibility that compliance professionals share and that help set them apart from others in the corporate environment.

The first level of responsibility is duty to the public.[21] This makes it clear that the compliance professional's job is more than just performing the employer's work. This is an element that characterizes any true professional. The standard of performance is not intramural, and is not determined by the next memo from one's supervisor.

The standards also emphasize that the compliance professional is not just an advisor, or one who can sit by passively after delivering advice to management. The compliance professional has an obligation to use whatever resources are available to interdict misconduct. Thus, for example, the compliance officer might advise that a proposed course was improper. The manager who received this message might elect to disregard it. At that point the compliance officer would have to escalate the issue to higher levels in the organization. But the compliance officer would not stop with a memo that received no response. He or she would keep on the issue, using whatever arguments and tools were available to win the point. At this stage, for example, it could become very important that the compliance officer have the ability to downgrade other managers' evaluations for that year, and have unlimited access to the board of directors and an audit committee. There is much more to the picture than giving advice once and then retreating. Compliance professionals are not just advisors; they are "players" or agents in the process of preventing misconduct.

The second level of responsibility set out in the standards is the most obvious one, at least on the surface—the duty to one's client or employing organization.[22] As an employee and as a compliance professional, the compliance officer and others in the program have a duty to perform at their professional best. They have duties of loyalty, confidentiality, and competency.

But the duty to the client can also come with some surprises. The duty is not owed to the managers of the business, nor is it a duty to follow what is in the short-term interests of those managers. The compliance professional has a duty to serve the long-term interest of the company, and this should always equate to compliance with the law. Thus, a compliance professional may be forced by this duty to interdict activities even of the chief executive, and raise issues with the board if necessary to prevent wrongdoing.

The compliance professional also owes the client organization the duty to perform at a high level of competence, even if this is not what management wants. Thus, a compliance professional will decline to conduct an investigation with limits imposed that interfere with the ability to conduct the investigation correctly.

The third level of responsibility is to the compliance profession.[23] This may strike some as an abstract notion, but it is key for the future of compliance professionalism. This responsibility reinforces the other two areas of responsibility. By following standards of competency and independence, the compliance professional helps ensure that future clients will get what they are paying for when they retain a compliance professional.

CONCLUSION

The government has given strong impetus to the development of effective compliance programs in organizations. As part of this initiative, government and the legal system have increasingly offered preferred treatment to companies if they accept the new model of the good citizen corporation. This good citizen is one that engages in steps to prevent and detect misconduct, voluntarily discloses the misconduct, and takes steps to remedy the misconduct.

Although there is much information available about the systems that can be used to develop effective programs, there can be no question that it will be the people who implement and monitor these programs who will make the difference. If there is a professional group of practitioners charged with this responsibility, then this experiment with voluntary compliance programs holds out great promise, both for the companies who employ these practitioners and for the society that benefits from having effective corporate self-policing.

The compliance professional is not just old medicine in a new bottle. This new position differs from other corporate functions in significant ways. It is these differences that help ensure that compliance professionals will establish a lasting place in modern organizations committed to being good citizen corporations.

NOTES

1. U.S. SENTENCING GUIDELINES MANUAL ch. 8 (1993).

2. U.S. SENTENCING GUIDELINES MANUAL § 8A1.2, comment (n 3(k)(2)) (1993).

3. U.S. SENTENCING GUIDELINES MANUAL § 8A1.2, comment (n 3(b)) (1993).

4. *See, e.g.*, Department of Health & Human Services, Office of Inspector General, *Compliance Program Guidance for Hospitals*, 63 Fed. Reg. 8,987 (1998).

5. In re Caremark Int'l Inc. Derivative Litigation, 689 A.2d 959 (Del. Ch. 1996).

6. Burlington Indus., Inc. v. Ellerth, 524 U.S. 742 (1998); Farragher v. City of Boca Raton, 524 U.S. 775 (1998).

7. Kolstad v. American Dental Ass'n, 527 U.S. 526 (1999).

8. HEALTH CARE COMPLIANCE ASSOCIATION, CODE OF ETHICS FOR HEALTH CARE COMPLIANCE PROFESSIONALS, R2.2, Commentary (1999).

9. *See* J. KAPLAN ET AL., COMPLIANCE PROGRAMS AND THE CORPORATE SENTENCING GUIDELINES: PREVENTING CRIMINAL AND CIVIL LIABILITY 16.57 (1993 & Ann. Supp.).

10. *Do the Corporate Sentencing Guidelines Require a Narrow and Legalistic Approach?*, 4 CORP. CONDUCT Q. 24 (1995).

11. W. Swenson & N. Clark, *The New Federal Sentencing Guidelines: Three Keys to Understanding the Credit for Compliance Programs,* 1 CORP. CONDUCT Q. 1 (Winter 1991).

12. *See* D. DRISCOLL ET AL., THE ETHICAL EDGE: TALES OF ORGANIZATIONS THAT HAVE FACED MORAL CRISES 105 (1995).

13. *See,* for example, the standards of the Department of Justice for antitrust compliance programs, *in* N. Roberts, *Antitrust Compliance Programs under the Guidelines: Initial Observations from the Government's Viewpoint,* 2 CORP. CONDUCT Q. 1 (1992).

14. *See* Chapter 3, *A Model for the Compliance Professional: Consulting, Policing, and Managing.*

15. U.S. SENTENCING GUIDELINES MANUAL § 8A1.2, comment (n 3(k)(7)) (1993).

16. HEALTH CARE COMPLIANCE ASSOCIATION, CODE OF ETHICS FOR HEALTH CARE COMPLIANCE PROFESSIONALS, R3.1, Commentary (1999).

17. *See* Chapter 3, *A Model for the Compliance Professional: Consulting, Policing, and Managing.*

18. In re Caremark Int'l Inc. Derivative Litigation, 689 A.2d 959 (Del. Ch. 1996).

19. R. Goldstock, *IPSIG: The Independent Private Sector Inspector General Program,* 4 CORP. CONDUCT Q. 38 (1996).

20. HEALTH CARE COMPLIANCE ASSOCIATION, CODE OF ETHICS FOR HEALTH CARE COMPLIANCE PROFESSIONALS (1999).

21. HEALTH CARE COMPLIANCE ASSOCIATION, CODE OF ETHICS FOR HEALTH CARE COMPLIANCE PROFESSIONALS, Principle I (1999).

22. HEALTH CARE COMPLIANCE ASSOCIATION, CODE OF ETHICS FOR HEALTH CARE COMPLIANCE PROFESSIONALS, Principle II (1999).

23. HEALTH CARE COMPLIANCE ASSOCIATION, CODE OF ETHICS FOR HEALTH CARE COMPLIANCE PROFESSIONALS, Principle III (1999).

CHAPTER 3

A Model for the Compliance Professional: Consulting, Policing, and Managing

Christine Parker

INTRODUCTION

The U.S. Sentencing Guidelines for Organizations requires a compliance program to meet seven standards,[1] which necessitates that the compliance professional must juggle—at least potentially—the following variety of professional roles and skills.

Standard	*Professional Roles and Skills*
"The organization must have established compliance standards and procedures to be followed by its employees and other agents that are reasonably capable of reducing the prospect of criminal conduct."	*Legal Knowledge, Risk Assessment and Management, Management System Design*
"Specific individual(s) within high-level personnel of the organization must have been assigned overall responsibility to oversee compliance with such standards and procedures."	*Senior Management Authority, Performance Assessment, Receiving Direct Reports, Information Management, Advocate for Compliance*

I would like to thank Simson Chu for diligent research assistance; Angus Corbett for useful discussions; Joseph E. Murphy, Jan C. Heller, and Neill Buck for helpful comments on a draft of the chapter; and all the compliance professionals I have interviewed for their insights.

"The organization must have used due care not to delegate substantial discretionary authority to individuals whom the organization knew, or should have known through the exercise of due diligence, have a propensity to engage in illegal activities."	*Human Resources Management, Investigation*
"The organization must have taken steps to communicate effectively its standards and procedures to all employees and other agents (e.g., by requiring participation in training programs or by disseminating publications that explain in a practical manner what is required)."	*Training, Advising, Coaching*
"The organization must have taken reasonable steps to achieve compliance with its standards (e.g., by utilizing monitoring and auditing systems reasonably designed to detect criminal conduct by its employees and other agents and by having in place and publicizing a reporting system whereby employees and other agents could report criminal conduct by others within the organization without fear of retribution)."	*Policing, Investigating, Auditing, Monitoring, Managing and Acting on Reports, Complaints Handling, Hotline Operator, Handling Whistleblowers*
"The standards must have been consistently enforced through appropriate disciplinary mechanisms, including, as appropriate, discipline of individuals responsible for the failure to detect an offense."	*Investigations, Policing, Discipline and Human Resources Management*
"After an offense has been detected, the organization must have taken all reasonable steps to respond appropriately to the offense and to prevent further similar offenses—including any necessary modification to its program to prevent and detect violations of law."	*Systems Review, Management Consulting Advice, Conducting Root Cause Analyses, and all of the above roles*

Given these standards, it is not surprising that role conflict and role ambiguity are a common experience for compliance professionals.[2] Compliance professionals are hired to act as a bridge between the requirements of law and ethics, and the internal culture, management, and strategic direction of their organizations. This means that compliance professionals must be nimble and flexible in helping managers and employees, reforming and operating management structures, being tough on wrongdoing, and negotiating with regulators. The design and implementation of an effective compliance program requires compliance professionals to fulfill a kaleidoscope of roles, exercise a variety of talents, and be skilled at multiple aspects of management. They should be able to combine those skills with an exhaustive knowledge of law, regulatory practice, and company policy; and be able to predict what are likely to be the major risks and issues of the future to which regulators, investors, customers, and public interest groups might hold the organization accountable.

This chapter argues that most of the compliance professional's tasks and skills fit into three major roles: (1) consulting, (2) policing, and (3) managing. The consulting role requires the ability to catalyze change and empower others to comply. The policing role ensures compliance through monitoring, enforcement, and correction. The managing role embeds compliance in daily operations, practices, procedures, and planning.[3]

This chapter sets out the objectives and limits of each role, when it is appropriate to play each role, and how compliance professionals should relate to management and employees of the organization in each role. These roles may also conflict, and sometimes one role will fit more comfortably in the organization than others. However, each is incomplete without the others. This does not mean that every individual compliance professional must play all three roles simultaneously all the time. The different roles will usually be shared around a compliance team and in-house legal department, or between an internal compliance officer, in-house attorneys, and external consultants and auditors hired for specific jobs. Effective compliance design backs up each role with the others in a holistic compliance program.

CONSULTING: CATALYZING CHANGE AND EMPOWERING OTHERS FOR COMPLIANCE

The first major role that compliance professionals must play is one of consulting, whether they are in-house or external professionals. Here the role is that of an active, engaged advisor—to the board, to management, and to individual employees. The consulting compliance professional is not aloof and independent, but is an active participant in the organization's business and culture as change agent, coach, and conscience. The key skill in the consulting role is to match information about the standards of the outside world (rules, laws, public perceptions, social issues) with indepth knowledge and experience of the inside world of the organization's business and management. The compliance professional has "one foot planted firmly in the shifting, treacherous terrain of the law, and the other planted just as firmly in the oozing swamp of business."[4] It is, then, the compliance professional's role as consultant to prompt internal organizational change, from the board level all the way down to the individual employee, with vision and fresh ideas about how to respond to external compliance risks and opportunities.

In the consulting role the compliance professional has the following tasks:

- Objectively (and continuously) identifies compliance risks and opportunities by knowing the organization's business intimately and by identifying the laws, regulations, and codes of practice, as well as trends in public opinion, consumer preferences, and investor policies on organizational responsibility, that might impact on the business.
- Prompts organizational change by identifying compliance solutions and opportunities and "selling" them to senior management.
- Empowers people for compliance by training, coaching, and advising managers and employees on preventive compliance and responses to breaches.

The compliance professional is charged with being the "conscience or consciousness of the firm" by the chief executive officer (CEO) and senior management. It is the job of compliance professionals to stay aware of the external environment, including laws, rules, codes of practice, perceptions of ethics, and changing values, and the compliance risks they pose to their employing organization. It is also compliance professionals' business to transform and prevent shortsighted organizational processes that ignore external legal and social responsibilities. As consultants, compliance professionals prompt change and coach members of the organization on compliance. They do not attempt to fulfill all the organization's compliance requirements themselves. A compliance unit with scores of staff is probably trying too hard to do all the compliance themselves, and is not taking the consulting element of the compliance role with enough seriousness. Paradoxically, an organization that appears to support compliance with lots of resources for its compliance staff may not take compliance seriously where it really matters in culture, commitment, and capacity throughout the whole organization. It is the consulting role to assist others to perform compliance. Compliance involves persuading the organization to change, beginning with senior management and moving through the whole organization.

As change agent at the senior management level, the compliance professional's consulting role involves building compliance commitment and capacity through an ongoing task of focusing senior management's attention on compliance risk, then building commitment by envisioning compliance as an essential strategic issue for the business. To "grab senior management attention," the compliance professional constantly stays aware of new laws, rules, regulatory practices, and issues that might affect the organization, and then communicates them to management, emphasizing the threat of legal sanctions and bad publicity, as appropriate.[5] Effective compliance professionals are powerful internal advocates for compliance. They tell stories of the risks of noncompliance, liability, and publicity disasters that have faced competitors and the employing organization itself in the past, to compel management to recognize the need for an active compliance management strategy.

It is in the next step that the real ingenuity, skill, and vision lies. The most imaginative compliance professionals convince their companies to see compliance not as a grudging response to potential penalties and industry standards, but as a source of strategic opportunities for business value enhancement. The "business case" for building a commitment to compliance can incorporate the savings, the marketing opportunities, the possibility to enhance reputation and legitimacy, or the need simply to keep up with commonly held views of good business practice that compliance brings. The best compliance consultants lead their senior management to look "objectively and dispassionately" at all their legal requirements and simultaneously find ways to turn compliance into a market advantage or as a means to increase efficiency. This requires "vision, leadership, commitment, lateral thinking, and imagination."[6]

The evidence shows that the organization that can harmonize compliance and business to achieve regulatory and business goals simultaneously can do better at compliance *and* business.[7] The compliance professional as consultant must offer business solutions, not just prohibitions—an equitable workplace that attracts excellent staff and that has minimal paperwork and prohibitions; a plant with a good reputation with workers and local communities; and satisfied, well-informed consumers. A recent study on construction firms that had experienced a worker death divided them into: (1) those that several years after the event had responded "virtuously" by re-evaluating organizational safety levels, altering workplaces or work practices, and re-emphasizing current safety policy; (2) those that had displayed a "blinkered" response limited to isolating and altering those visible and specific factors that led to the particular death in question; and (3) those that displayed no change.[8] The data showed that those firms that displayed a virtuous response also had a "virtuous culture."[9] A virtuous culture was one that saw "safety as integral to organizational activity, while the culture lacking in virtue would tend to push safety into the background in order to focus on short-term demands."[10]

The compliance professional's consulting role flows from being a change agent at the senior management level, to helping upper and middle management accommodate compliance demands in daily business, to communicating compliance standards and procedures to employees and agents through training, advice, and practical help at the grassroots level (of course, in practice these different roles will often overlap at all three levels of the organization). On a daily basis, business managers and employees want compliance professionals who "understand and focus on business objectives," who "don't say no" but who offer solutions and find ways to legally achieve business goals. Compliance professionals are expected to act as consultants who "facilitate business objectives" by being "service providers, not decision makers."[11]

> The compliance people who have been the most successful are the ones that don't go around beating up on business units. They keep commercial reality in their minds. . . . They are the ones with the gentle approach who get business on their side. . . . Good compliance people have enough business acumen not to be too theoretical, but to give solutions. Otherwise you just have clashes all the time.[12]

Effective compliance professionals describe it as a "marketing exercise" to be visible and accessible to all employees. They make themselves available through hotlines, frequent visits to the sites where people actually work, and a friendly, helpful demeanor. They will help employees with any problems they have so that employees, in turn, have confidence to come to them with compliance problems. Their aim is to educate ordinary people in business to take ownership and responsibility for compliance themselves. Therefore, compliance professionals spend much of their time trying to change the behavior and attitudes of employees and managers by training employees in standard operating procedures that embed compliance in the organization. They also try to engage employees' values to change attitudes toward compliance.

In summary, the strengths of the consulting role are in prompting organizational commitment and capacity to change for improved compliance, binding compliance to the business and strategic goals of the organization, and empowering others to comply. If the consulting role is done well, the compliance professional might find him- or herself out of a job. This will never happen in reality, of course, because as soon as one compliance risk is faced and addressed by one part of the organization, there will always be a new risk that the compliance professional must identify and help the organization address somewhere else. The consulting role should be the first role of the compliance professional, because without it, the compliance program will not get past square one.

However, the consulting role cannot be the only role for the compliance team. At some point an effective compliance professional needs to have the management authority to follow through on compliance issues. A compliance professional who cannot monitor and investigate whether the compliance policy is followed, nor impose a compliance decision on a line manager when necessary, will be completely ineffectual. Empowering and catalyzing compliance are essential, but so too are policing and managing.

POLICING: ENSURING COMPLIANCE THROUGH MONITORING, ENFORCEMENT, AND CORRECTION

The second role that the compliance professional must undertake is policing. Ultimately, most organizations hire compliance professionals not just for advice, but also for assurance that the organization is meeting its compliance obligations. Even excellent consulting functions are of little use if the board and senior management have no idea whether appropriate compliance performance is actually being achieved within the organization. Compliance professionals must police compliance in order to identify and rectify compliance breaches speedily. This is generally the least popular element of compliance work, but also the most crucial, because managers and employees will never know if all the other compliance activities are accomplishing anything if someone does not police compliance. The policing role is concerned with knowing and responding to compliance breaches before they become regulatory disasters or publicity nightmares. It is a protective system than can detect failure in the organization's management systems, and the very existence of policing functions can discourage noncompliance and sloppy practice.

The policing role includes the following tasks:

- *Monitoring* involves concurrent oversight of whether the processes that make up the compliance program are being implemented and are functioning as designed (for example, by monitoring attendance at training programs, the level of implementation of standard operating procedures designed to improve compliance, and employee feedback on implementation of the compliance program); and of the level of compliance; that is, how often and where compliance violations are occurring (for example, by checking employees' paperwork, the number of accidents or compliance incidents, the level of complaints, and whether the compliance program matches new laws and compliance risks). This often requires the introduction of systems to ensure that the compliance manager receives information about compliance breaches (for example, through hotlines (and other procedures to protect anonymity of whistleblowers), complaint-handling systems, reports from line managers about compliance incidents, and informal conversations with managers and employees).

- *Auditing* entails after-the-fact evaluations conducted periodically to check that compliance efforts are effective, including onsite visits, interviews with personnel, and reviews of written materials and documentation.

- *Investigations* require designing and coordinating internal investigations of suspected compliance violations (discovered through monitoring, auditing, regular management reports, complaints, and/or hotlines), and recommending corrective action.

- *Reporting* necessitates providing the results of monitoring, auditing, and investigations to the board of directors and senior management with recommendations for action, discipline, and sanctions; and also coordinating the reporting of self-discovered violations to regulators where disclosure is necessary or advisable to take advantage of voluntary disclosure policies.

- *Evaluations/Review of Organization's Compliance Performance* involves putting all of the above together to evaluate the compliance program's implementation and effectiveness, sharing assessments with senior management, and recommending corrections and enhancements.

To perform the policing role, the compliance professional needs independence from line management and from those being investigated or audited. The compliance professional also needs authority to access and review all documents and areas of the organization relevant to compliance activities. The level of independence required will vary from task to task, with the need for independence greatest in periodic full-scale audits (perhaps annually), and in investigations of serious large-scale wrongdoing (especially where a large number of employees or members of senior management may be involved). It is important that auditors and investigators always be sufficiently independent so as to be insulated from any pressure asserted by those being audited or investigated. In some cases, external auditors or investigators should be hired to ensure that independence is preserved, and is seen as being preserved. It is always advisable for the compliance professional to report directly to the CEO and Board Audit or Compliance Committee on audits and investigations. The policing compliance professional will be independent of line managers in conducting audits, investigations, and monitoring, but will share responsibility with senior management, including human resources, for deciding on and implementing solutions, sanctions, or management changes in response to self-discovered compliance breaches. The compliance professional and the organization may also incur external reporting obligations if they discover something that the law requires to be disclosed, especially if it affects public health or safety.

The strength of the policing function is in ferreting out weaknesses, asking hard questions, and imposing requirements on the business, but all with a view to protecting the long-term performance of the organization. However, compliance teams that do nothing but police organizational compliance and enforce the rules quickly lose trust and cooperation with both management and employees. Who wants to cooperate with a policeman? Where is the vision in monitoring and auditing? Thus, the policing role must be connected to the consulting role to remain relevant to business goals and strategies, to envision change, and to stay connected to employees' values and concerns. Although the consulting role catalyzes and empowers compliance culture, it has no authority to enforce compliance. The policing role catches and corrects breaches once they have occurred. But a compliance team that uses only consulting and policing roles lacks any system for ensuring compliance on a daily basis. It is daily management of compliance that holds the whole thing together. The policing role is useless if there is no day-by-day monitoring and implementation of compliance controls.

MANAGING: EMBEDDING COMPLIANCE IN DAILY OPERATIONS, PRACTICES, PROCEDURES, AND PLANNING

The third role that the compliance professional must assume is that of compliance management. Here the compliance professional is a partner in the management structure of the organization. He or she is not just an advisor, catalyst, or coach, but rather an integral member of the management team. He or she does not act as monitor, enforcer, or prosecutor, but rather as designer, guide, and problem solver, with the aim of making compliance a natural and easy part of everyday operations. The management role is the nuts and bolts of preventive compliance programs; it "embeds" compliance in the management, culture, and goals of the organization. The key skills that the compliance professional needs to exercise in fulfilling this role are to understand how to use management systems, operating procedures, reward systems, and reporting structures to guide and motivate people to comply; and to effectively manage information about compliance coming from disparate points within the organization to identify where compliance is an issue. This is a role that is shared with other managers. In this role, the compliance professional needs the support and backup of the rest of the management team in order to exercise "clout," authority, and respect so that compliance will "trump" self-interest and negligent noncompliance at the points where it really matters.

As Driscoll, Hoffman, and Murphy point out, the consulting (catalyzing and empowering) function and the management function may seem inconsistent at first, but they are really essential supports for each other:

> It is true that buy-in by all employees is a key objective of any program, but there is still a need for specific managers to participate in a more detailed way and take responsibility for the pro-

gram. Here there is an apt analogy to the company's internal auditing function. Every employee in a company is responsible for financial integrity, but it is still recognized that a separate internal auditing group is needed to give this focus and direction and to serve as a check on the process. So, too, compliance managers serve a similar purpose.[13]

Compliance managing is about designing operating procedures and management systems for preventing breaches before they occur, and managing people and information for compliance on a daily basis. It includes the following tasks:

- matching risks, laws, and regulations to relevant businesses, units of operation, and individual job descriptions in order to make it clear which roles and units need to comply with which provisions and principles; including competence and skills analysis to identify the compliance tasks and responsibilities of every individual in the company
- designing management structures, standard operating procedures, directives, and guidance systems to ensure that managers and workers comply with the identified provisions—this might include operating system redesign, product redesign, requirements on which designated individuals periodically "sign-off" to indicate that they have fulfilled certain compliance requirements, compliance performance reporting requirements, new standard operating procedures, and changed job profiles and decision-making criteria for investments that include compliance criteria
- assisting in assessments of managers and employees that include compliance performance assessment
- backing up all the above with discipline and rewards for individual and unit compliance performance to motivate employees and managers toward compliance as evaluations, rewards, and potential discipline drive the rest of business conduct
- receiving and acting on information from direct reports, complaints, hotlines, informal conversations, and reviews and evaluations on how to continuously improve the compliance program and compliance performance of the organization

Good compliance programs are ultimately about management ingenuity.[14] They are a challenge of creativity, politics, and understanding of human motivations. The good compliance manager knows what will motivate people to comply. He or she works with managers to put incentives, sanctions, procedures, systems, and equipment in place to facilitate maximum compliance. These systems push the responsibility for compliance onto every worker and manager as a natural part of their jobs. They "cascade" responsibility for compliance down through line management, so that line managers work with compliance managers to ensure compliance. The compliance professional's first management job will often be the design of compliance management systems. For example, standard operating procedures might specify when and what protective clothing should be worn, safe procedures for operating machinery, what information should be given to customers or investors before completing a transaction, which documents should be checked by attorneys, what events should trigger a report to compliance, and so on. In factories this could also include equipment design that makes noncompliance impossible or difficult, technology that reduces or avoids pollution, safety barricades, automatic shutdowns, and so forth. In services industries, analogous efforts to prevent noncompliance by design can be accomplished by computerized systems. For example, some securities houses use computerized systems that will not allow traders to complete trades that would breach conflict-of-interest rules, capital maintenance requirements, and other rules.

In designing compliance management systems, good compliance managers listen first. They spend time learning the corporate culture and identifying risky situations that are likely to arise. They aim to be helpful and look for commercially viable solutions to compliance problems, rather than laying down inflexible rules and then walking away. Compliance managing therefore builds on the compliance consulting role. The aim is that compliance professionals and the systems they produce are "embedded" in the management, culture, and goals of their organization, as influenced by the organization as by legal values and regulatory goals.[15]

Compliance management then puts compliance into organizational planning. Central strategic planning must set positive goals for compliance performance. One of the main aims of a compliance program is to incorporate compliance issues into internal decision-making agendas. Compliance must be part of the central coordination and accountability functions of the organization if middle managers and employees are to take it seriously. This means that compliance must be a senior management "corporate" function, not just a sideline at middle management level. Excellent compliance functions make sure compliance goal setting and informed decision making about investment in compliance self-regulation are an integral part of top-level corporate strategy and planning.

Effective compliance managers will also use incentives and sanctions to achieve desired employee conduct. Studies of correlates of illegal behavior in organizations have found that organizations that have in place both (1) clear standards and expectations about inappropriate behaviors, and (2) reward systems to monitor and reinforce expectations, probably reduce compliance breaches.[16] In another study, Pastin and Brecto, business ethics consultants, concluded from their sample that poor ethics compliance environments correlated significantly with performance measures or reward systems that employees saw as attaching financial incentives to behavior inconsistent with ethical conduct.[17] Positive motivators are also an essential part of an effective compliance management program, especially in any organization that uses incentives and evaluations as an integral way to achieve its other objectives, such as sales and productivity targets, or quality control. There is no reason in principle why compliance performance should be any harder to evaluate than other employee traits such as leadership or the ability to develop subordinates.[18]

Compliance professionals assist line managers to design and implement appropriate compliance management procedures, but then give much of the responsibility for day-to-day management of compliance to the ordinary management chain. However, the effective compliance manager will continue to receive and analyze information about the daily operation of the compliance program through:

- regular direct reports from managers on whether compliance procedures have been followed and on any compliance issues that arise
- queries and concerns reported through the employee hotline
- external complaints handled by the complaint-handling staff
- informal conversations with people
- information received via the compliance policing function, that is, monitoring, auditing, and investigations

The special skill of compliance professionals as managers is one of management of information: using information about the daily operation of the management system to determine when to step back into active compliance management.[19] The compliance professional as manager will understand what events trigger the need for active compliance intervention in the form of rectification, discipline, a positive incentive or reward, a challenge to a line management decision, or the need for a wider decision about policy and procedure. Therefore, compliance managing involves an information-sifting role. It involves looking for patterns and indications of problems and knowing when compliance needs to move into active compliance management, and not just letting line managers operate the system. Compliance professionals therefore must be part of an adequate information dissemination and reporting system within the organization.

Both evaluative studies of what makes corporate self-regulation effective and compliance managers' own folklore find that compliance professionals' political resources, status, and clout within an organization make a significant difference to effectiveness in management functions. Although independence is very important in the policing role, it is clout and authority that are most important in the management role because it is in the management role that the compliance professional must have the authority to challenge decisions and implement procedures, sanctions, and rewards. In his study of corporate crime in the pharmaceutical industry, Braithwaite concluded that one of the conditions for making corporate self-regulation work was ensuring "that pro-public interest constituencies within the corporation are given organizational clout."[20] In this context, Braithwaite suggested that examples of strengthening clout for pro-public interest constituencies would include:

[G]iving the international medical director an unqualified right to veto any promotional materials from a subsidiary which do not meet corporate standards of full disclosure of product hazards, having the plant safety officer answerable to a head office safety director rather than subject to the authority of the plant manager whom s/he might need to pull up for a safety violation, having quality control independent from marketing or production pressures, [and] having an international compliance group answerable only to the chief executive officer.[21]

Most professionals who have worked in compliance managing know that

. . . clout is everything. If you assign compliance to an individual in the organization who is not well-regarded, or who does not exercise independent management responsibility, or is viewed in reality as a lackey or subordinate for some other real agenda that everyone knows about, you cannot expect satisfying results from your compliance function. From the earliest stages of the compliance initiative in the organization, executive management at the highest levels must express its unconditional commitment to and seriousness about compliance—and must vest in the selected CO [compliance officer], unconditional responsibility and authority to address the issue as it rolls out throughout the organization.[22]

In practical terms, clout means that line managers and employees know from experience that the compliance professional's advice is likely to be backed up by senior management and that if they go against it, they are likely to be overruled.

[T]he CEO's signature and pictures of his or her smiling face on compliance policies are not enough. Only a history of support for compliance in the face of crunch contests between line managers and compliance staff is convincing evidence that the compliance policies will not be discounted according to the philosophy of "watch what the bosses do, not what they say."[23]

Clearly the best way to achieve clout is through the direct support of the senior management, preferably of the CEO personally.

In summary, the managing role is the nuts and bolts of compliance. It holds together the two other elements—consulting and policing. Management builds on consulting by moving compliance into daily action to prevent breaches. It supports policing by implementing sanctions, rewards, and management changes to address self-discovered breaches. This does not mean that one person has to do everything. Within a compliance unit, there may be those who specialize in each of the separate roles. The legal department will quite likely provide some of the compliance consulting advice (for example, keeping abreast of legal risks), as will external consultants, auditors, or investigators who may be hired in from time to time.

CONCLUSION

The smart compliance team uses consulting, policing, and managing to weave together a robust web of compliance—one that is strong on adding value to business goals, strategies, concerns, and values; strong on embedding in daily management practices and motivations; and strong on assurance that risks are covered and that if something goes wrong, then the organization will know about it before the regulators or the public do. The consulting role convinces managers and employees that compliance is in everyone's long-term interest and builds compliance credibility for moments when tough action must be taken. The policing role ensures that compliance is not just good words and good intentions, but a tough protection against the risks of liability, enforcement action, and negative publicity. The management role puts consulting visions and ideas into practice, and addresses and corrects the weaknesses identified by the policing role.

Each organizational compliance team will need people with personal and professional commitment to leadership on legal and social responsibility values; the ability to champion compliance through a combination of leadership, strategic thinking, value-adding, and political influence; a deep understanding of how to motivate and manage; and the skill of asking hard questions politely but firmly. But remarkable personal and professional skills are not enough; compliance professionals must also enjoy appropriate institutional support, including direct access to and communication channels with all areas of the organization, senior management support to win employee commitment, and the ability to escalate conflict up the chain of command quickly to where it can be appropriately addressed. It is only with these skills and supports that compliance professionals will be able to effectively use their kaleidoscope of roles to protect and support their employing organizations.

NOTES

1. The seven standards presented here are the *minimum* elements required to qualify an organization for the possibility of mitigation in sentencing under the Guidelines. U.S. Sentencing Commission, *Sentencing of Organizations*, U.S. SENTENCING GUIDELINES MANUAL ch. 8 (1992). For a discussion of how these apply to health care compliance programs, *see* T. Bartrum & L.E. Bryant, *The Brave New World of Health Care Compliance Programs*, 6 ANNALS OF HEALTH L. 51–75 (1997). *See also* P. Fiorelli, *Fine Reductions through Effective Ethics Programs*, 56 ALB. L. REV. 403–40 (1993); J. KAPLAN ET AL., COMPLIANCE PROGRAMS AND THE CORPORATE SENTENCING GUIDELINES (1993 & Ann. Supp.).

2. In a preliminary survey of occupational stress among U.S. health care compliance officers, Heller and Guetter concluded that they were "more likely than most professional groups to experience stress associated with workload, role conflict, and role ambiguity." *See* J.C. Heller & J.R. Guetter, *Is Compliance Officer a Tough Job, or What?*, 1:3 J. HEALTH CARE COMPLIANCE 45–50 (1999).

3. The term "embedding" comes from B. Sharpe, Making Legal Compliance Work (1996).

4. Here the commentator was describing the similar role of general counsel. T. Terrell, *Professionalism as Trust: The Unique Internal Role of the Corporate General Counsel*, 46 Emory L.J. 1005–10 (1997).

5. *See* J. Murphy, *Selling Compliance to Management: 10 Sales Tips*, 9:13 ethikos (July/Aug. 1999).

6. B. Dee, Compliance: Where It's Been, Where It is Now, Where It is Heading?, Address at the Association for Compliance Professionals of Australia Annual Conference Dinner, Sydney, Australia (May 29, 1997).

7. *See, e.g.*, M. Porter & C. van der Linde, *Green and Competitive: Ending the Stalemate*, Harv. Bus. Rev., Sept.–Oct. 1995, at 120–34; J. Mathews, *More Innovative Workplaces = Safer Workplaces: Organisational Innovation and the Protection of Workers' Health and Safety*, 13:4 J. Occupational Health & Safety—Australia & New Zealand 319–29 (1997).

8. F. Haines, Corporate Regulation: Beyond "Punish or Persuade" 69 (1997).

9. F. Haines, Corporate Regulation: Beyond "Punish or Persuade" 123 (1997).

10. F. Haines, Corporate Regulation: Beyond "Punish or Persuade" 94–95 (1997).

11. L. Cotton, Compliance Theory and the "Real World," Presentation to the Second Annual Conference of the Association for Compliance Professionals of Australia (1998) (notes of the presentation are on file with the author).

12. Interview with a compliance professional for a research project on Corporate Compliance and Corporate Citizenship (September 19, 1998). *See* C. Parker, *Compliance Professionalism and Regulatory Community: The Australian Trade Practices Regime*, 26:2 J. L. & Soc'y 215–39 (1999).

13. D.M. Driscoll et al., *Business Ethics and Compliance: What Management is Doing and Why*, 99 Bus. & Soc'y Rev. 35–51 (1998).

14. *See* B. Sharpe, Making Legal Compliance Work (1996).

15. B. Sharpe, Making Legal Compliance Work (1996).

16. *See* T. Mitchell et al., *Perceived Correlates of Illegal Behaviour in Organizations*, 15 J. Bus. Ethics 439–55 (1996). Mitchell et al.'s study was based on the perceptions and experience of human resources directors in 31 electronics firms. It is one of the most reliable and comprehensive studies on this topic available and reviews previous studies on the topic.

17. M. Pastin & C. Brecto, *The Impact of Corporate Ethics and Compliance Practices: A Survey*, 3:4 Corp. Conduct Q. 51–54 (1995). Note that the authors of this study did not report the same stringent reliability and validity tests on the data from their sample as scholarly authors usually do.

18. J. Murphy, *Evaluations, Incentives and Rewards in Compliance Programs: Bringing the Carrot Indoors*, 3:3 Corp. Conduct Q. 40–43 (1994).

19. I am indebted to Mr. Angus Corbett, Senior Lecturer, Law Faculty, University of New South Wales, Sydney, Australia, for this point.

20. J. Braithwaite, Corporate Crime in the Pharmaceutical Industry 302 (1984).

21. J. Braithwaite, Corporate Crime in the Pharmaceutical Industry 302 (1984).

22. H. Zinn, *Some Organizations Call It "Compliance Officer"—Some Call It "Designated Felon": Considerations in Designating, Empowering and Supporting your Organization's Compliance Leader*, 1 Corp. Compliance 533–47 (1999 PLI).

23. J. Braithwaite & J. Murphy, *Clout and Internal Compliance Systems*, 2:4 Corp. Conduct Q. 52–53 (Spring 1993).

CHAPTER 4

Evaluating the Compliance Officer

Winthrop M. Swenson

INTRODUCTION

In the last decade, the field of compliance management has moved from exotic to mainstream. Studies show that the U.S. Sentencing Guidelines for Organizations, and other policies such as the Department Health and Human Services (HHS) Office of Inspector General (OIG) Guidances, have prodded most leading organizations to formalize their management of compliance. Despite the strength of this trend, one of the surest ways to instill a "deer in the headlights" expression on the face of an otherwise self-assured chief executive officer (CEO) or board member is to ask what seems like a fundamental question: How do you *know* that your compliance program is working?

To be sure, some members of senior management do not think much about this question. They live in a state of peaceful denial, assuming that because they *personally* have integrity, compliance or ethics problems cannot happen at *their* organization—notwithstanding evidence that this may be wishful thinking.[1] Even among these optimists, however, the pointed question, "But how do you *know* that your program is effective?" seems to create some pause. The fact is, most CEOs are ill equipped to answer this question.

A closely related but, as will be shown, *not* identical question is the topic of this chapter: How do you know if your compliance officer is doing a good job? Amazingly, although compliance officers have become fixtures in many organizations, this also remains a question that most organizations have difficulty answering. The confusion is bad for organizations and, although some compliance officers may take a "don't-rock-the-boat" comfort in the fuzziness of their evaluation process, the truth is, this is bad for compliance officers as well.

It is understandable that organizations struggle with the topic of how to evaluate the compliance officer—it comes with plenty of challenges. And, because organizations vary in key respects, there is no "one-size-fits-all" method that will work for every company. To find the right approach, each organization must recognize the challenges and develop a plan for evaluating the compliance officer that makes sense for that particular organization. On the other hand, although tailoring is key, there appear to be principles that can guide the process of settling on a specific evaluation approach. This chapter discusses these guiding principles and the challenges that give rise to them.

WHAT IS AT STAKE?

Before pondering these guiding principles, it is important to recognize why getting this right is so important. It boils down to this: creating a thoughtful process for evaluating the compliance officer greatly improves the odds that the organization will actually achieve the benefits that a compliance program can offer. Why is this so? When organizations go through the process of developing a meaningful approach to evaluating the compliance officer—let alone undertaking the actual evaluation—they invariably undertake critical thinking about the program's objectives, the roles and responsibilities of those responsible for making the program work (*not* just the compliance officer), and metrics for demonstrating program success.

This exercise, in turn, not only makes the program more effective, it puts the organization in a position to demonstrate to the government, if the need should ever arise, that its program is worthy of "credit." The organization can show this because the organization itself has come to a coherent understanding of why such an assertion would be true. In contrast, experience has repeatedly shown that when an organization has not gone through this process, its program is less apt to be effective and the organization is less likely to be persuasive in explaining why its program is a good one.

Developing a sound approach to evaluating the compliance officer also has important resource implications. First, the process of evaluating the compliance officer helps the organization identify its compliance priorities. When an organization understands its compliance priorities, it can more efficiently target its scarce compliance resources. Second—and this must be stressed as one of the key reasons compliance officers should welcome the development of an evaluation process—evaluating the compliance officer, if done well, helps management understand what the compliance officer is being asked to accomplish. This often leads to more realistic budgets for compliance officers, more accountability for others whose support is needed for compliance success, and a more significant role for the compliance officer within the organization. On the other hand, a poorly conceived approach to compliance officer evaluation can do more harm than good. Consider these two differing evaluation examples and the pitfalls associated with each.

Example A. Company A's compliance officer reports to the board of directors on initiatives he has undertaken in the last year, and the board is impressed. "We updated and reissued our code of conduct," he explains during a 20-minute presentation. "We completed both companywide training on sexual harassment and targeted training on antitrust. Calls to our help line have steadily declined, which shows that concerns about compliance are diminishing. No serious allegations warranting investigation have come to light. Recent auditing in certain compliance-sensitive areas revealed no significant issues." Pressed to stay on schedule with a packed agenda, the board thanks the compliance officer for a very good year's work and moves on to consideration of an important bond offering. The compliance officer receives a comfortable raise and bonus.

However, the board does not know that although the actions that the compliance officer has taken in the last year sound good, a closer look at the quality of these initiatives would leave a different impression. The code of conduct was updated, but many supervisors failed to distribute it and talk about it to employees as planned. Employees considered the antitrust training they received, which explained what was required with legal terms like "with intent to restrain commerce," to be confusing. As for the apparently good "results" from the program, there has been no recent effort to re-publicize the help line and employees who have used it have felt that they did not get a quick response. One employee even felt that her supervisor knew that she had used it and was hostile as a result. These impressions have percolated around the organization and are the main reason for the reduction in help line calls.

The audits that were done were superficial and reflected the auditors' lack of understanding about "real world" compliance issues associated with the risk areas that were audited. In one part of the organization, serious ethical problems are occurring with clinical trials financed by a pharmaceutical company. Although employees there are afraid to raise their concerns with management, one has already complained to a government watchdog that, unbeknownst to the organization, is preparing to investigate.

Example B. The board of directors of a large municipal hospital has received a report that two of its businesses may have engaged in illegal cross-referrals of patients. The matter is still being investigated, but to make matters worse, recent "look forward" audits of billing practices show no improvement in the recent training of staff charged with billing responsibilities. The board directs the general counsel to give the compliance officer a "needs substantial improvement" rating when he conducts the compliance officer's performance evaluation.

However, the board does not know that the executives in charge of the units involved in cross-referring patients are known to be highly—some would say, overly—aggressive, and they resisted training on the organization's code of conduct in their units. The allegations of cross-referrals came to light through the Integrity Advice Line, which is the only compliance program feature that the compliance officer has been able to develop and publicize without interference. The compliance officer had tried to raise her concerns about the pushback she was getting from the business unit directors, but the general counsel was unwilling to take on these executives. The chief financial officer (CFO) approved the content of the billing training over the objections of the compliance officer, who believed it was poorly designed.

These two examples illustrate a range of issues that can arise in evaluating the compliance officer. The most fundamental and controversial is whether it is ever fair or appropriate to evaluate the compliance officer in terms of the *impact* that the program appears to be having on compliance. The first example illustrates the dangers of *not* seeking to gauge the program's impact. Here, the steps the compliance officer has undertaken, and various other superficial indicators, effectively mask fundamental weaknesses. The board thinks all is well and it is not. Another compliance officer doing a much better job of executing could have given the same report and the board would have been unable to tell the difference. By failing to look at impact, the board is really in the dark as to which type of performance it has gotten. These considerations argue in favor of including impact measures in the compliance officer's evaluation.

The second example seems to cut exactly the other way. Here, the board had some indication of the program's impact but the results misled the board about the *compliance officer's* job performance. In fact, where the compliance officer had the authority to act—for example, in setting up the Integrity Advice Line—she seems to have done an effective job. The Advice Line successfully surfaced issues about which the organization needed to know. Thus, by tagging the compliance officer with the program's negative results, the board is not being fair or accurate in assessing the compliance officer's work.

So which approach is right? Is it appropriate to look at a compliance program's impact in assessing the compliance officer's job performance? If the answer is, "It depends," then, what factors help resolve the uncertainty? What about new programs that are just beginning, or ones that are being significantly revamped? Would it ever make sense to look at a compliance program's impact while the program is undergoing such change? If program impact is not the "be-all-end-all," what else is relevant in the evaluation of a compliance officer?

THREE WINDOWS ON MEASURING PERFORMANCE: DESIGN, IMPLEMENTATION, AND IMPACT

It has recently been proposed that there are three ways to evaluate the effectiveness of a compliance program: by looking at the quality of the program's design, the thoroughness of its implementation, and the actual impact that the program is having.[2] By extension, this same evaluation approach can be applied to evaluating the compliance officer's effectiveness. However, as the two examples earlier and the discussion that follows make clear, the approach must be carefully tailored to the realities of a particular compliance officer's circumstances. This basic "three window" evaluation approach is not complex. It can be described as follows.

Design. Evaluating the compliance officer's performance from the design standpoint means assessing whether the compliance functions that the compliance officer is responsible for creating are sufficient. Sufficiency can best be thought of in terms of applicable governmental pronouncements such as the U.S. Sentencing Guidelines and HHS OIG Guidances; and best practices that similarly situated organizations have generally found to be effective. If the design of an organization's compliance program meets these criteria, it is safe to say that the compliance officer has done his or her job from the design perspective; the program should satisfy the government and it reflects the best available thinking about what makes programs work.

Implementation. Having the right design for the program is a good start, but many programs fall short because the plan is not fully executed. Tasks that are supposed to be accomplished, in fact, are not. The second window, then, looks at the compliance officer's "follow-through" in carrying out the plan's directions. If the design meets best practice standards and the follow-through is complete, the program can be thought of as *presumptively* effective.

Impact. The third potentially relevant way of evaluating the compliance officer's performance is by gauging the program's actual impact. Sometimes the question is asked, because impact would seem to be the truest indicator of the program's success, why not look at *just* impact? One answer is that measuring impact is a complex task. To comprehensively measure a program's impact really requires a huge number of separate evaluations. For example, learning that employees in one business unit are following procedures for compliance with the Toxic Substances Control Act does not mean that employees in another business unit are doing so, and it tells you even less about whether employees in either unit are willing to trust the company's system for reporting sexual harassment complaints, which is practically a requirement to fend off equal employment opportunity (EEO) liability.[3]

The range of issues that potentially could be tested to evaluate the impact of a compliance program is too great to rely on impact testing alone. A more realistic approach is to rely on the presumption of effectiveness that a best practices design and thorough implementation provide, and then use resource-intensive impact measures to selectively test effectiveness in higher priority areas.

There is, however, a way to expand the reach of impact testing without unrealistically straining resources. To explain this concept, it is useful to draw a distinction. What does it mean to test impact? The most obvious way is to undertake "transaction auditing"; in other words, to look directly at actions by employees that involve compliance issues and check to see if things were actually done right. In health care, this can work for billing and coding by pulling the relevant physical records. Financial services companies can look at cash transactions to see if the required cash transaction reports (CTR) were filed when dollar amounts so require it. Utilities can look at interactions between affiliates to see if steps required by affiliate rules are being followed, and so forth. But how do you "audit" to see if sexual harassment is occurring? What about antitrust, where misconduct is likely to be oral? And what kind of transaction auditing is possible to see if sales personnel are unethically misleading customers? For some kinds of compliance risks, traditional concepts of auditing are difficult to apply, if not impossible.

Moreover, it has already been pointed out that it would be a fool's errand to try to audit *every* compliance risk that exists within an organization, especially in a large, diverse organization where audit findings in one part of the business may not accurately predict conduct, even within the same risk area, in another part of the business. Finally, today's suspected compliance risk—the one for which the company audits—may not be the compliance headache that actually materializes tomorrow. Did Bankers Trust suspect that misappropriation of escheated funds would lead to a major settlement with banking authorities? Did Sears think that it would have to deal with a criminal case involving violations of bankruptcy laws? Did the U.S. Army see the sexual harassment trouble coming several years ago when the tip of that iceberg first began to surface? Because compliance breaches can be difficult to predict, transaction auditing also suffers in that it may generate a false sense of security about how effective the overall compliance program is.

A second way to gauge impact comes at the idea more indirectly. Instead of testing actual compliance in specific risk areas, the idea behind this approach is to test the quality of the *systems* on which the organization is relying to *prevent, detect,* and *respond* to violations, both the general systems that cut across all risk areas (for example, the help line) and systems within the organization's specific risk areas. On the prevention side, for example, evaluate whether employees find their training (general code of conduct and specific-risk, such as antitrust) to be relevant, understandable, and consistent with what the organization is asking them to do in other aspects of their job (that is, it is not being overridden by revenue, budget, or schedule pressures). With respect to detection, find out if the help line has a healthy call volume and whether employees say that they would trust talking to their supervisor or calling the help line about an ethical issue. Information in this latter case would have helped the board in Example B above understand that the compliance officer was doing what she could do well.

How to undertake indirect impact testing is discussed later in this chapter, in the section Evaluation Tools or Strategies. Suffice it to say here that when an organization has a basis for believing that its various compliance-supporting systems are working well, it has a basis for believing that its overall compliance program is effective. This indirect, systems-oriented approach to evaluating impact can then be augmented by direct, targeted transaction audits to further test compliance in areas of higher perceived risk.

APPLYING THE "THREE-WINDOW" APPROACH TO THE COMPLIANCE OFFICER'S EVALUATION

The description of the three-window evaluation framework provides an overview of what *can* be looked at in evaluating a compliance officer, but what *should* be? Keeping in mind the misleading impressions created by Examples A and B, what actually is fair and appropriate? The principal factors that influence the answer to this question are the maturity of the program and the "jurisdiction" or actual responsibilities of the compliance officer.

Maturity of the Program—Allowing the Evaluation Approach to Evolve

As a general principle, the less developed or immature a program is when the compliance officer is tasked with running it, the more the compliance officer's initial evaluation should emphasize program design. This stands to reason. If a program needs a lot of work before it will have the basic features of best practice compliance programs, the compliance officer's main task is building up the program. At the outset of this process, the emphasis therefore should be on design, and the evaluation should consider whether the compliance officer is planning the right components to make the program a creditworthy, best practice program.

Because formal evaluations typically occur annually and the design of even a full-scale program can largely be done in well under a year, it is fair to say that the first formal evaluation should also include significant implementation considerations. Here, the evaluation should consider whether the compliance officer is completing the steps called for under the plan in a timely and thorough manner. Over time and subject to the job "jurisdiction" considerations described below, the compliance officer's evaluation should shift more and more toward impact (with relatively little emphasis on design, except as new program features are added, and modest emphasis on implementation, which typically will become increasingly routine "maintenance"). The emphasis should increasingly shift, in other words, to the question of whether the systems the organization is relying on to prevent, detect, and respond to violations (and for which the compliance officer is responsible) are effective.

"Jurisdiction"—What is the Compliance Officer's Job?

The question of what the compliance officer is responsible for is critically important. By mid-2000, the Ethics Officer Association (EOA) had more than 700 members.[4] The titles of the professionals making up EOA vary widely from "Chief Compliance Officer" to "Director of Business Conduct" to "Vice President of Ethics" and more. Titles can mislead, but the fact is that the actual jobs of these professionals vary, too.

Some compliance officers are tasked primarily with operating the hotline, and many are assigned this function along with responsibility for distributing and developing training around the code of conduct. Under this model, subject matter experts—who do not report to the compliance officer—are responsible for managing compliance (for example, risk assessment or training) within particular risk areas. Other compliance officers have much broader responsibility, sometimes virtually everything described in the U.S. Sentencing Guidelines' "seven steps" (except, often, auditing), including overall management compliance in all risk areas.

Example B showed that it is unfair to hold a compliance officer accountable for compliance activities that fall outside the compliance officer's duties. A first step, then, in deciding how to apply the "three window" evaluation framework to the compliance officer is to determine the aspects of the program over which he or she actually has control. The compliance officer should be accountable for the design, implementation, and impact of those aspects of the program for which he or she has responsibility—and no more.

The Critical Question—Whose Job Is Compliance?

In deciding for what the compliance officer is responsible, there are really two considerations—one straightforward, one less so. The first is whether a compliance area or system falls, in a formal sense, within the compliance officer's job description. For example, many organizations carve out a compliance area and assign that area to a subject matter expert other than the compliance officer. If that is the case (for example, the human resources department conducts all training on EEO issues), then the compliance officer should not be responsible for the design, implementation, or impact of that training. Drawing these kinds of boundaries is not difficult.

The second consideration, which is harder but critically important, is whether some other person may be in a position to influence the nature or impact of something that is within the compliance officer's job description. The issue most often comes up with respect to impact measures, and especially direct measures of compliance where, after all the training and messaging by the compliance officer is said and done, an employee may still do the wrong thing because his or her supervisor cared more about a short-term revenue target than about doing things "the right way." Going back to Example A, a factor that may have reduced the effectiveness of the help line is that a supervisor appeared to have retaliated against an employee for using it. In example B, unit heads undercut the compliance officer's efforts, at a minimum with respect to compliance training, and probably more broadly than that.

All of this underscores a well-documented fact about compliance. It is not a one-person job. A recent study found that the top three reasons cited by employees for misconduct that they had observed were (1) cynicism about whether the compliance messages were real, (2) pressure to meet schedules, and (3) pressure to meet budgets.[5] Cynicism is often a product of supervisors telling employees, at least implicitly, "This is not what's really important around here." Schedule and budget pressures are typically well beyond the ability of a compliance officer to control. If these kinds of forces are at work in a company, surely the compliance officer should not be tagged for the negative compliance results or "impact" that they may generate.

Finally, compliance is, in the end, everyone's job. A real risk here is that an organization will buy into the idea that impact is relevant in assessing the compliance officer, but apply the principle in a simplistic way (as happened in Example B). Employees in any organization of size *will*, at least occasionally, make mistakes—the compliance officer's job is not to make sure that this never happens, but rather to take reasonable and diligent actions to reduce the risk that it will happen.

The Dilemma of the Non-Expert Evaluator

To add one more level of complexity, most members of senior management or boards—the people typically charged with performing compliance officer evaluations—are not terribly sophisticated about compliance. This is no slight to their intelligence, it is just that this is a field with its share of complexities and managers often have a limited understanding of them (although sometimes they may think that they know more than they do!). Troublesome evaluation processes like those in the two earlier examples happen all the time, and they happen because those responsible for evaluation do not know better. To avoid such results, organizations need a means to educate management on how to conduct compliance officer evaluations appropriately.

In sum, then, the "three window" evaluation framework is useful, but consideration must be given:

- To where the program is in the developmental process. This will influence the right mixture of design, implementation, and impact measures that should comprise the evaluation at any one moment in time. In general, the earlier in the developmental process the program is, the more the compliance officer's evaluation should center on design and implementation; the more mature the program is, the more the evaluation should consider impact.
- To the compliance officer's formal responsibilities and the ability of others to influence his or her duties, especially when assessing program impact, but potentially also (as Example B illustrated with the roll-out of training) implementation.
- To a strategy for educating evaluators on how to evaluate. This can be politically awkward because the evaluators may not recognize their own ignorance in this area.

EVALUATION TOOLS OR STRATEGIES

With these principles in mind, the evaluation options can be summarized as described in Table 4–1.

With respect to assessing the compliance officer's performance on design, there are three options. The first really contemplates taking a "pass" on including design performance in the compliance officer's evaluation, that is, not because the program is already mature and well developed

Table 4–1 Evaluation Options

Evaluation "Window"	Tools/Techniques	Outside Help?
Design	Compliance Officer credentials	No
	Process Report	Maybe
	Gap analysis	Yes
Implementation	Audits, interviews	Maybe
Impact		
Direct (transaction testing)	Targeted compliance audits	Maybe
Indirect (systems evaluation)	Employee survey, focus groups, specialized feedback	Desirable, especially for surveys and focus groups

(which would be a separate and legitimate reason for downplaying design in the evaluation), but because of the compliance officer's recognized expertise. Some compliance officers are hired into the position because of their knowledge of the organization's business but do not have substantial experience in the compliance field. However, others are recruited precisely because of their compliance experience—either generally, or with respect to risk-specific compliance (for example, billing in health care, anti–money laundering in financial services). For those hired because of their experience, it may be entirely appropriate to assume that they can competently design the basic program elements for which they are responsible. Their compensation should reflect that expertise, but their evaluation should focus on follow-through (that is, implementation) and impact over time.

A second option is to have the compliance officer map a step-by-step strategy for developing the program's design, and then to evaluate the compliance officer in terms of a self-report on his or her completion of the steps called for by that strategy. For example, the compliance officer may decide that step one in this design strategy is to outline categories of activity that must be accounted for in the compliance program (for example, elements of the U.S. Sentencing Guidelines' "seven steps"); the next step is to execute a game plan for identifying best practices within each system category (for example, attend Health Care Compliance Association and

Ethics Officer Association meetings, interview six peer organizations with mature programs to understand their programs in detail); and the final step is to synthesize this information into an overall compliance plan. The compliance officer can then prepare a "process report" for the evaluator, summarizing the steps taken and how the design has emerged from them.

This approach can provide the evaluator with a standard against which to measure performance, that is, steps undertaken pursuant to a plan that appears logical on its surface; but its weakness is that the evaluator probably lacks the experience to gauge whether a plan that "appears logical on its surface" is, in fact, a good one, or whether the design that has emerged from it is sufficient. This is the dilemma of the above-discussed non-expert evaluator.

A potentially more reliable, third approach is to retain outside help from a seasoned compliance consultant. A consultant can use a best practices "gap analysis" (essentially a model that distills, in detail, the elements of a best practice compliance program) to assist in the evaluation of a compliance officer in either of two ways. First, the consultant can take an "after the fact" role and review the proposed plan the compliance officer has developed to provide feedback on whether the plan reflects best practices. Another, more team-oriented approach (see further discussion, On Supportive Consultants and Realistic Goals) involves the consultant from the outset. The consultant works with the compliance officer to develop best practice parameters for the compliance program's design and the compliance officer completes the process, conferring with the consultant on an as-needed basis. The outcome of this approach is this: the evaluator has a credible, defensible basis for evaluating the compliance officer's design performance, provided by the consultant's feedback, but the compliance officer is set up to win, because he or she has had the benefit of the consultant's feedback along the way.

The key in selecting a consultant is making sure that the consultant understands how to assist in the evaluation process. The consultant also should have a credible gap analysis approach and the experience in the field to back it up (unfortunately, quite a few consultants have entered the field with rather limited resumes). Experience should include general knowledge of compliance best practices and an understanding of compliance requirements in any technical areas where the organization has significant exposure. Best results are often obtained when individual consultants team together (for example, an expert in compliance generally teams with experts in coding, environmental health and safety, or whatever the organization's salient risk areas are).

Evaluating the compliance officer on implementation is conceptually straightforward. The program design calls for specific tasks to be undertaken; the goal here is to ensure that they have been completed. The first step, then, is to map the program. The evaluator needs to understand key features of the plan that are expected to drive success. If the compliance program's design or plan is not documented in reasonable detail—and many compliance program plans are not—this may require the evaluator (or his or her designee, see below) to sit down with the compliance officer to obtain this understanding. Once the key facets are understood, the evaluator (or, again, the designee) can undertake an evaluation to see how well implementation has taken place.

Coming back to the job jurisdiction issue, it is critically important that the evaluator understands the limits of the compliance officer's responsibility for, and ability to, implement the program. In Example A, all supervisors did not distribute the company code of conduct. But was this the compliance officer's responsibility? Depending on how the organization has assigned roles and responsibilities, the answer might be "Yes" or it might be "No." The answer might be "Yes" from the responsibility perspective. It was within the compliance officer's contemplated responsibilities to verify that code distribution/training occurred. But it might be "No" from an accountability standpoint, because she had no ability to influence the unit executives' actions. (In the example, the compliance officer was unable to persuade the general counsel to take action, and no other avenues of recourse were apparent.) These kinds of questions must be appreciated and understood.

Techniques for evaluating implementation include auditing, in the sense of checking to see that required events (for example, specified procedures for a hotline, code training at orientation, and planned risk-based training) are occurring. Interviews with personnel in a position to know about required compliance activities are a logical part of the process as well.

Realistically, if the evaluator is a high-level person in the organization, he or she may want to assign this implementation verification to someone else. Internal Audit may be a logical candidate, but once again, this is an area where an experienced outside consultant can be of possible assistance. In addition to the general benefit of bringing a measure of credibility to the process, an independent evaluator may be able to better appreciate some of the important nuances that are relevant to this undertaking; these include a better "feel" for what is worth checking into and the previously mentioned job jurisdiction issues that can come into play in sorting out any implementation shortfalls.

With respect to impact, the available tools correspond to the two ways impact can be gauged: directly and indirectly. With respect to direct measures, transaction audits can be used to test actual compliance in areas where such testing is possible and where, given the resources required to undertake transaction auditing, the risks are relatively greater.

With respect to indirect measures, again the goal is to evaluate the strength of the systems on which the organization is relying to prevent, detect, and respond to misconduct. On prevention, for example, the organization wants to be sure that employees understand the company's core values as well as their specific compliance responsibilities (for example, antitrust, sexual harassment, or conflicts of interest) that relate to their jobs. The organization also wants to ensure that supervisors and senior management are perceived as supporting compliance; otherwise, when all is said and done, compliance may well be overridden by a belief that "this isn't what really matters here." On the detection side, the organization wants people to believe that a "shoot the messenger" mentality does not prevail, and that they can raise issues with supervisors or through the help line with confidence.

If one were to rely on only one tool to gauge the strength of compliance systems (and, as will be discussed, one tool is not recommended), by far and away the single best tool is an employee survey with benchmarking capabilities. Benchmarking in this context means an ability to compare an organization's individual results with average results from comparable organizations. Benchmarking is critical because if the compliance officer is going to be assessed on impact in any way, a realistic point of comparison is key. For example, one of the factors known to influence the willingness of employees to raise compliance/ethics issues is fear of retaliation. If an organization probes this issue on a survey and determines that 30 percent of its employees are not sure whether they might experience retaliation, is this a good result or a bad one? The availability of a benchmarking database helps answer the question.

Surveys that have been designed with impact evaluation in mind have these benefits:

- *Surveys offer the most efficient means of obtaining a measure of compliance system strength throughout the organization.* It has recently been proposed[6] that one way to visualize the way a compliance program operates is to see its activities functioning in a multitude of distinct "cells." Each cell represents the intersection of one of the organization's array of risk areas (for example, government contract compliance), one of its distinct compliance systems (for example, training), and a particular business unit where compliance is expected to be achieved. A well-designed survey can extract effectiveness information with respect to general compliance impacts (for example, do employees believe senior management strongly supports compliance, does the organization treat help line calls confidentially) but also in these particular cells (do employees (1) in the Southside Division find (2) the environmental compliance (3) policy manual clear and understandable; do employees (1) in the Home Health unit understand (2) the antitrust (3) training they have received).

- *Surveys help disentangle the "whose job is it, anyway?" question.* If a survey's sample size has been designed to be large enough, data will be available from individual business units. By comparing results among business units, it becomes easier to determine whether any weaknesses in results (for example, lack of confidence about retaliation in reporting misconduct) are systemic, and therefore arguably more likely to be the compliance officer's responsibility, or specific to particular units, and therefore more likely to derive from things supervisors are doing in those units. This kind of information can be extremely illuminating in helping the evaluator understand that others in the organization influence compliance—*not* just the compliance officer—and in bringing about the accountability needed to make the program run more effectively (for example, creating survey-based performance measures for business unit heads, fostering constructive discussions between the compliance officer and business unit heads about how to solve issues, and so forth).

- *Surveys help identify compliance program priorities that, in turn, help set achievable performance goals for the compliance officer and others.* A requirement for effective evaluation of the compliance officer is being able to set specific and achievable goals. Because surveys present a coherent picture of the "cells" where compliance activities occur, priorities for future action naturally emerge. These priorities can be easily converted into goals for the compliance officer and others charged with compliance program responsibilities.

Surveys are definitely the purview of outside experts. As of this writing, KPMG's Integrity Managing Services (developed with input from Walker Information, a company that has itself developed ethics-related survey instruments)[7] and the Ethics Resource Center[8] have developed surveys with benchmarking capabilities that can be used for evaluation purposes of the kind described here. The KPMG instrument permits greater evaluation detail.

Two other impact-related tools can be used to complement surveys and transaction auditing: focus groups and what might be called "specialized feedback." Focus groups can be an excellent way to obtain qualitative insight "from the trenches" on compliance issues, especially to further explain results from an employee survey where the results are necessarily somewhat general. Although valuable in this respect, focus groups arguably may be better used as a diagnostic tool to help the compliance officer design compliance strategies, rather than providing yet another source of information for the evaluation. There are two reasons this may be the case. First, conducting focus groups is a specialized science/art, generally requiring outside assistance. Second, and more important, information gleaned from focus groups is qualitative; that is, it can help explain what drove the results of a survey, as noted, but it is not necessarily generalizable to the entire organization. In short, focus group information may not be "hard" enough on which to pin an evaluation.

Specialized feedback can, in contrast, be critically important to the evaluation. It comes into play when the compliance officer has important duties that the other impact evaluation techniques (that is, transaction auditing, employee survey) are not helpful in analyzing. In some organizations, for example, the compliance officer may be charged with conducting investigations, the performance of which cannot easily be tested through the other impact measures. Here, those in position to judge the compliance officer's work—perhaps the general counsel with respect to investigations—should work with the compliance officer to develop performance metrics and then participate in the evaluation process to assess success against those metrics.

The compliance officer may have some unusual duties where this approach will require modification. For example, some compliance officers have as an important assigned duty the obligation to work cooperatively with regulators. These regulators cannot, realistically, be expected to help set performance metrics for the compliance officer, but they can be interviewed to determine how well they think the compliance officer is performing this aspect of his or her job. In this particular example, such a meeting (for example, by a board member and regulatory personnel) would have the additional benefit of reinforcing the idea that the organization cares about the regulators' views.

Specialized feedback will be necessary when—before a compliance officer can even turn to designing and implementing a compliance program—he or she faces immediate "triage" duties. In other words, some compliance officers are hired amid, or in the aftermath of, a compliance crisis. In this kind of situation the compliance officer's duties may entail putting out various kinds of fires, for example, helping develop evidence for litigation-related discovery requests, rapidly developing and deploying policies related to the crisis, and/or conducting root cause analyses and investigations. This may mean, in turn, that formal goal setting is impractical, and that after-the-fact discussions with those in the best position to evaluate the quality of the compliance officer's contribution will be the sole means of evaluation.

ON SUPPORTIVE CONSULTANTS AND REALISTIC GOALS

Throughout this discussion, the option of retaining an outside consultant has been noted. The fact is, there is a healthy role outsiders can play in the success of a compliance program. Nowhere is this truer than with respect to the topic of evaluation. As noted, potential benefits of using a consultant in the evaluation process include:

- *solving the problem of the "non-expert evaluator"*—A third-party consultant can provide the knowledge necessary to ensure not only a meaningfully rigorous evaluation, but also one that is realistic and fair for the compliance officer.
- *helping the organization recognize that compliance is not a one-person job*—It can sometimes be difficult for the compliance officer, particularly in the early stages of building or rebuilding a program, to make the "job jurisdiction" argument (discussed earlier) that others (for example, business unit heads, legal staff) have responsibility for the program, too. A neutral outsider can help educate the organization about this critical point that, in turn, can make the evaluation of the compliance officer fairer and the accountability of others more likely.

• *injecting independence and credibility*—A consultant with recognized expertise can imbue the program with credibility in precisely the areas most likely to be critically scrutinized by the government; namely, the questions of the organization's commitment to compliance and the program's actual effectiveness.

This said, the use of a consultant can be uncomfortable and counterproductive for both the organization and the compliance officer if the consultant is seen not as a supportive partner, but rather as a "gotcha" adversary. To avoid this result, the consultant ideally should be brought into the goal-*setting* process. For example, the organization and compliance officer can work with the consultant to create a baseline on employee perceptions regarding facets of the existing program through an employee survey, and then identify specific, achievable goals toward which the compliance officer ought to strive going forward. A re-administration of the survey can be used to measure success. If the consultant has expertise in these kinds of surveys (for example, has a benchmarking database against which to interpret results), the goals should be attainable and the result is therefore a "win-win" situation. The evaluation sets real and important goals, and the compliance officer successfully meets those goals.

Whether a consultant is utilized or not, as with any goal-setting/evaluation process, goals should be as specific and achievable as reasonably possible. Some of the evaluation techniques discussed readily lend themselves to this objective (for example, implementation "audits" to verify follow-through) while others (for example, special feedback from a regulator), because they are inherently somewhat subjective, will make this objective more challenging.

DOCUMENTING SHORTCOMINGS

The main premise of this chapter is that carefully—and knowledgeably—considering the performance of the compliance officer yields important dividends. Essentially, it helps enable the compliance officer to operate effectively, because it creates an informed understanding of his or her job function, and this, in turn, makes the compliance program itself more effective. This said, evaluation of the compliance officer (just as is the case with evaluation of the overall program) entails some risk. Evaluations typically suggest areas for improvement (at least implicitly and most often explicitly), and what might be intended as a constructive suggestion in the context of a performance evaluation could be cast as an admission of program inadequacy in the context of adverse litigation. This risk should not be overstated. Real world examples of evaluative information being used against a company that used the information constructively (that is, to strengthen the compliance program as opposed to, for example, covering up the information) are exceedingly rare. Moreover, the government has increasingly been sending the signal that evaluation of program effectiveness is critical to a company receiving "credit" for its compliance program.[9] This said, prudent steps can be taken to minimize exposure to this litigation risk; these include limiting the degree to which sensitive information is written down and taking steps to establish attorney/client and work product privileges (for example, have the evaluator report to counsel) with respect to the communication of particularly sensitive information.[10]

CONCLUSION

The process of evaluating the compliance officer is one for which there is no one "right way." The characteristics of the compliance officer's job, the specific risk areas confronted by the organization, and other factors, make it necessary for organizations to find their own approach. Along the way, the principles discussed in this chapter can provide guidance. Despite the challenges, developing a meaningful approach to evaluating the compliance officer is well worth the effort. Properly accomplished, far from undercutting the compliance officer, it should generate understanding and support for the compliance officer and, through a number of secondary effects, strengthen the overall program.

NOTES

1. *See* KPMG Integrity Management Services, 2000 Organizational Integrity Survey, which found a high incidence of observed misconduct among respondent employees (76% reported observing misconduct in the prior year) and a common perception that management is often in the dark (57% agreed that their CEOs and other senior management "do not know what type of behavior goes on in the company").

2. *See* W. Swenson et al., *Measuring the Effectiveness of Compliance and Ethics Programs, in* COMPLIANCE PROGRAMS AND THE CORPORATE SENTENCING GUIDELINES—PREVENTING CRIMINAL AND CIVIL LIABILITY (1993 & Ann. Supp.), which presents a version of the model described here.

3. *See* Faragher v. City of Boca Raton, 524 U.S. 775 (1998).

4. Ethics Officer Association, <http://www.eoa.org/general.htm>.

5. *See* KPMG Integrity Management Services, 2000 Organizational Integrity Survey.

6. J.M. Kaplan, *Thinking Inside the Box: Risk Analysis in Three Dimensions,* 14 ETHIKOS 1 (Sept./ Oct. 2000).

7. KPMG, Integrity Managing Services, 2000 Organizational Integrity Survey, <http://www.us.kpmg.com/services/content.asp?l1id=10&l2id=30>.

8. Ethics Resource Center, 2000 National Business Ethics Survey, <http://www.ethics.org/2000survey.html>.

9. For a discussion of government pronouncements stressing the necessity of program evaluation, see W. Swenson et al., *Measuring the Effectiveness of Compliance and Ethics Programs, in* COMPLIANCE PROGRAMS AND THE CORPORATE SENTENCING GUIDELINES—PREVENTING CRIMINAL AND CIVIL LIABILITY (1993 & Ann. Supp.).

10. For detailed discussion of these risks and the potential use of privilege, see A. Valukas et al., *Threshold Considerations, in* COMPLIANCE PROGRAMS AND THE CORPORATE SENTENCING GUIDELINES—PREVENTING CRIMINAL AND CIVIL LIABILITY (1993 & Ann. Supp.).

CHAPTER 5

Thinking Like a Compliance Professional: The HCCA Code of Ethics for Health Care Compliance Professionals

Mark E. Meaney

INTRODUCTION

On January 28, 1986, Jerald Mason of Morton Thiokol asked his vice-president of engineering to think like a manager and not like an engineer. Robert Lund, the engineer, acquiesced, and a few hours later, millions watched in horror as the space shuttle Challenger blew up in the Florida sky, killing all seven astronauts on board.

The pressure had been tremendous. NASA wanted to launch the shuttle. Congressional support for the shuttle program was on the line. A final draft of the President's State of the Union address awaited news of the first teacher in space. At first, Lund had refused approval for the launch. It was simply too dangerous. If one of the defective "O-rings" failed in flight, the shuttle could explode. Then, his boss said something that made him reconsider: "Take off your engineering hat and put on your management hat." Lund reversed his decision and approved the launch. The rest is history.

What separates "thinking like a manager" from "thinking like an engineer?" A code of professional ethics draws the line. When Mason asked Lund to think like a manager, he asked for more than Lund's approval. He asked Lund to disregard all that he knew to be true as an engineer. He asked him to think not in terms of his professional obligations and technical expertise, but in terms of the effect his decision would have on his boss, his company, NASA, Congress, and the President of the United States. Mason asked Lund to act as if he had never become an engineer.

The Challenger case demonstrates what can happen when a professional relies on personal beliefs in choosing how to practice his profession. The result was disastrous. Lund had failed to consider what an organization of. professional engineers has to say about what engineers should do in similar circumstances. Several formal codes of professional ethics provide engineers with clear guidance on what sort of behavior professional engineers ought to expect of one another. Specifically, engineering codes provide guidance on whether to weigh safety against the wishes of employers. Lund chose to rely on his own private judgment and give preference to his employer's wishes—and at what cost?[1]

Chapter 1 argues that health care compliance should be perceived as a profession in its infancy.[2] Health care compliance appears now to satisfy some, but not all, of the essential criteria that mark a profession. Health care compliance professionals (HCCPs) possess a high degree of skill and specialized knowledge; they are in the process of establishing their own standards and accreditation process to regulate entry into the field; and they perform an essential service to the community. The Health Care Compliance Association (HCCA) does not, however, have the state-enforced power to discipline members legally. The status of HCCPs as members of a profession, therefore, awaits the maturity of health care compliance as a practice both in relation to the law and to the health care system as a whole. Nonetheless, although society has yet officially to recognize health care compliance as a profession through state licensure, HCCPs should continue to be proactive in this regard. In short, HCCA should continue to develop the practice of health care compliance as a profession.

If HCCPs are to be proactive, they must recognize that members of a profession bear special ethical obligations toward society. An implied contract serves as the basis of these obligations. There is a kind of trade-off between society and the professions. In exchange for self-governance, members of a profession are expected to perform an important social function and serve the public good. Moreover, society depends quite heavily upon the integrity of the professions. Only members of a profession are truly competent enough to determine the qualifications of members. Because society entrusts professional associations with the regulation of the profession, society expects professional associations to set higher standards of conduct. Professional associations have the moral obligation to ensure that members live up to these standards. Partial fulfillment of this moral obligation begins with the formation, dissemination, and implementation of a code of professional ethics.

This chapter traces the development and dissemination of the new HCCA Code of Ethics for Health Care Compliance Professionals (Code). In particular, it focuses on the special relation of HCCPs to society. It begins with a general consideration of the nature and purpose of a code of professional ethics. It then briefly discusses the origins and development of the HCCA's Code. The final section suggests ways that HCCA might strengthen its commitment to professional ethical development through proper implementation of the Code. The Code represents only partial fulfillment of the association's moral obligations to society to set high standards of conduct for HCCPs. Although HCCA has begun the hard work of professional ethical development with the publication of the Code, much work yet needs be done.

THE NATURE AND PURPOSE OF A CODE OF PROFESSIONAL ETHICS

As suggested earlier, a code of professional ethics symbolizes an implied contract between society and members of a profession. Members of a profession are distinguished by the way that society accords them a greater degree of autonomy in the exercise of their authority than it does the trades, the arts, or business, because of the specialized nature of their skills and knowledge. Members of a profession establish their own standards and accreditation process, regulate entry into the field, and exercise a degree of self-policing. Such powers and privileges constitute a form of monopoly granted by society to members of a profession. In return, members of a profession are expected to perform an important social function and serve the public good. In a code of professional ethics, members of a professional association ought to acknowledge their social function and their commitment to serve the public good publicly.

A code of professional ethics also ought to reflect the special duties that follow upon the professional–client relationship. Chapter 1 draws a distinction between "customers" and "clients" to illustrate how members of a professional association ought to serve not only the public good, but also their own clients' good. Customers have the capacity to know what they need and to judge whether a service or a commodity satisfies those needs. Clients lack the requisite knowledge to diagnose their needs and to judge the proper means to the proper ends. It is argued that, although laypersons can judge certain aspects of the practice of members of a profession, clients are generally not competent to evaluate the quality of services rendered. Moreover, where a customer can criticize the quality of a commodity and perhaps demand a refund, clients must rely on experts to judge the competence of a member of a profession as well as to gain recourse in the event of malpractice. Trust thus serves as the foundation of the relationship between clients and members of a professional association.

Also, the relation of client to a member of a profession is more complex than customer to merchant. A businessperson is generally held to only the minimum moral standard of "do no harm" or "mitigate harm caused." Members of a profession, on the other hand, are held to a much higher standard. Members of a profession are expected to "pursue the good" of their clients. Consequently, professional codes of conduct ought to reflect the special nature of the obligation that members of a profession have to pursue the good of their clients.

Although a code of professional ethics is designed primarily to prescribe how members of a profession ought to pursue their common ideals of service to society and clients, it also solves a coordination problem. A code of ethics protects members from certain consequences of competition by making it more unlikely that other members will take advantage of their good conduct. If professionals can be confident that others will support them and protect them from the self-interested demands of clients, they are much less likely to accede to such pressures. A code of professional ethics thus also defines the manner in which members of a professional association ought to comport themselves in relation to each other. Professional associations are similar to unions in this sense, because they protect the interests of members. They are dissimilar, however, because individuals organize a professional association to help members serve others, while unions serve only the self-interest of members. Professional associations are thus similar in nature to charitable organizations or government agencies.

In summary, a code of professional ethics serves an important function. When a group of individuals in a similar occupation begin to organize as a profession, they normally draft a code of professional ethics in an attempt to begin to satisfy the social and ethical requirements of professionalism. As Joe Murphy argues in Chapter 2, professionals share a commitment to an ideal of service.[3] They organize to better serve the same ideal than they could if they did not cooperate. Chapter 2 also underscores the fact that an organized profession offers protection for members from certain pressures, such as the financial self-interest of clients. Thus, a code of professional ethics prescribes how professionals should pursue their common ideals by withstanding those pressures, so that each member knows how best to serve. In the final analysis, codes provide guidance for professional ethical development as well as a warrant for professional autonomy.

THE ORIGINS AND DEVELOPMENT OF THE HCCA CODE OF ETHICS FOR HEALTH CARE COMPLIANCE PROFESSIONALS

In 1998, the HCCA Board of Directors assigned the Education Committee the task of developing a code of ethics for HCCPs. The Education Committee subsequently asked Jeff Oak to chair the committee's Code of Ethics Task Force to draft the Code. The task force included Jan Heller, Joe Murphy, Jeff Oak, and Mark Meaney. Over the course of the next several months, the task force produced a working document, which was then forwarded to the HCCA Board of Directors for comment and distribution to members. After input from members was taken into account, the board approved the final draft of the Code of Ethics for Health Care Compliance Professionals in November 1999.[4]

In a series of preliminary teleconferences, the task force established some ground rules. They debated purpose, form, process, and content. First, they derived the aim or purpose of a professional code of ethics for HCCPs from the aim or purpose of a health care compliance program in general. Ultimately, a health care compliance program has its purpose to impact positively the quality of the delivery of health care to patients, residents, and clients, and to prevent fraud and other forms of misconduct. From these ends, it was agreed that HCCPs are stewards of public trust. HCCPs ought to use the Code to acknowledge this trust publicly and commit to high standards of professionalism, integrity, and competence. In short, the purpose of the Code is to identify and categorize those special obligations that HCCPs have to the general public, to employers and clients, and to the legacy of the profession.

Second, the task force settled on format. Form concerns the order of the parts to the whole. Generally speaking, there are two ways to approach the writing of a code: inductively and deductively. With an inductive format, authors determine the order of the parts to the whole in relation to the order of perceived importance of individual topics. For example, if the authors of a code of professional ethics think candor and trustworthiness more important than privacy and confidentiality, the authors place the former before the latter. Although this format has its virtues, the order of the parts to the whole can appear arbitrary to others. Moreover, codes with this format tend to be brief in nature and usually consist of a small list of statements that rarely have much structure at all. The task force agreed to adopt a deductive format. Here, authors use the end or goal of the code of ethics to deduce the relation of the parts to the whole. For purposes of logical rigor and clarity, this method seemed preferable.

If authors adopt a deductive format, there are then three models. First, some codes focus on principle. In a principles-based model, the order of the parts to the whole descends from a preamble or statement of intent and fundamental principles to canons and guidelines or commentaries. Second, some codes focus on relationships, in which case authors determine the order of the parts to the whole by the relative importance of relationships. For example, the relationship model usually begins with relations/obligations to the general public, followed by separate headings for relationships with employers, clients, and other members of the profession. Finally, a third model combines the principles-based model with the relationship model. For example, codes of ethics for health care professionals generally balance principles and relationships. They might begin with a preamble/statement of intent and fundamental principles, but they then generally focus those principles on relationships: obligations to the general public, the health care professional–patient relationship, and other members of the profession.

The task force chose to adopt the mixed model. They thought it appropriate to begin with a preamble/statement of intent and fundamental principles followed by rules and guidelines or commentaries. They also thought it important, however, to focus those principles, rules, and commentaries on the different kinds of relationships that HCCPs experience. HCCPs have responsibilities and obligations to the general public, to employers and clients, and to each other.

Third, the task force addressed process. They agreed that the process would consist of a number of stages. The four task force members would prepare a working draft of the Code. Once the preliminary draft was completed, the document would be submitted to the education committee and the board of directors for review and comment. They would also recommend to the committee and the board that the officers of HCCA give the membership every opportunity to review the draft carefully and critically. Because the writing of a properly functioning code of ethics is a collective task, the task force agreed that the process should include as much input from as many compliance professionals as possible. Without a reasonable amount of group consensus concerning standards of conduct relevant to the group, a code can end up "on the shelf" rather than embodied in the actions and decisions of members of the group. Moreover, a code of professional ethics should give substantial assistance to professionals who encounter unique ethical challenges. It should regulate the *actual conduct* of professionals and not merely list principles or unattainable ideals. Input from those professionals is therefore essential. The task force also looked at other professional standards and also drew on the preliminary work undertaken by an Ethics Officer Association committee.

The task force felt it was important, then, that the Code truly reflect collective agreements about relevant ethical issues by incorporating guidance from many quarters. To accomplish this end, the task force recommended to the committee and the board that they solicit input by circulating the preliminary draft and canvassing the membership for comment. The task force also felt that it would be helpful to get the reaction of professionals outside of the association, for example, from federal officials and health care attorneys. Thus, although it might prove difficult and cumbersome to reach consensus, it was agreed that this part of the process would produce the most effective code.

Finally, the task force reached preliminary agreement on the general nature of the content itself. It was felt that, if a code is to serve its purpose, then it should be specific and honest. It ought not merely to state in general terms that members should not lie, cheat, or steal. Professionals are in the best position to know how a member might abuse information and power without public awareness of their activities. Only those with comparable knowledge can best restrain unprofessional or unethical conduct on the part of practitioners. A professional code of ethics should therefore specifically address those areas that pose as special temptations to members. It should address those practices that, although not quite illegal, are nevertheless unethical. Specifically, it was agreed that the Code should address such areas as conflict of interest, discovery of wrongdoing, resignation, whistleblowing, retaliation, and confidentiality. Content is discussed in greater detail in the next section.

THE HCCA CODE OF ETHICS

As suggested, the task force adopted a deductive approach to writing the Code as opposed to an inductive approach. From the general aim or goal of a compliance program, the task force deduced the different parts of the whole. Then the parts were ordered by striking a balance between a principles and a relationship model. This means that the parts appear in a descending order from a preamble/statement of intent to general principles and rules to specific commentary, but that the principles, rules, and commentaries apply to relationships listed in order of importance.

The task force used an ideal of service to generate the general principles. The principles, in turn, ground the rules of conduct, and the commentaries make explicit the meaning of the principles and rules. Because HCCPs stand through their work in relation to the general public, employers or clients, and each other, the principles and rules were then applied to these relationships in that order. The Code not only identifies the principles and rules of conduct that should govern the behavior of compliance professionals, it also provides commentaries for guidance on the meaning and application of the principles and rules to these relationships. The commentaries thus make explicit how compliance professionals ought to apply the principles and rules; that is, they illumine specific areas of ethical concern.

The Preamble outlines the purpose of the Code. The claim is made that an HCCP's ideal of service encompasses a particularly vulnerable population. Moreover, the delivery of health care impacts not only patients and their families, but also ultimately the well being of the community. The assumption is made that the general public will judge the value of the work of compliance professionals by how it affects the delivery of health care. HCCPs are thus stewards of a public trust. This trust obliges HCCPs to uphold the highest standards of professionalism, integrity, and competence. The Code, then, publicly acknowledges the responsibilities of HCCPs to the general public, employers or clients, and the legacy of the profession.

Some HCCPs may have difficulty accepting this claim. After all, it may not be obvious to them how a compliance program impacts patient care, let alone the well being of the community. Some might argue narrowly that HCCPs have an obligation only to try to make certain that their employers or clients comply with the law. In response, without going too far afield, it could be argued that the Code was written with the assumption that, generally, the law is based on important societal values. For example, Medicaid/ Medicare rules and regulations play an important role in the just allocation of the nation's scarce medical resources and in protecting public funds. Of course, the allocation of medical resources has an impact, either directly or indirectly, on patient care. Compliance work therefore impacts patient care; its aim is a just allocation of the nation's scarce medical resources. Consequently, HCCPs' ideal of service encompasses not only patients and their families, but also ultimately the well being of the community. Compliance professionals also seek to ensure that the conduct of their employing organizations is ethical, that those organizations engage in fair and honest dealings with patients, and that they abide by other rules and societal values such as protection of the environment and protection of the health and safety of health care workers.

From this common ideal of service, the task force derived three principles. It was concluded that the most important relationship was that of HCCP to the general public or society at large. Naturally, this relationship includes the duty to comply with government regulations, but goes beyond the letter of the law to include an implied social contract or covenant between HCCPs and society. In the simplest of terms, the government agrees to provide financial reimbursement in exchange for the delivery of appropriate treatments and services to the most vulnerable members of society. It is important to note that children and the elderly receive the most in the way of government health care subsidies. The HCCP also actively seeks to promote the organization's commitment to law and ethics in the delivery of health care services directly to the public. In the relation of HCCPs to society, HCCPs in effect promise to uphold the public's trust in health service organizations, suppliers, billing companies, physician practices, and clinical laboratories. If any of these entities violate that trust, the HCCP has an obligation to resist.

The rules and commentaries listed under "Principle I: Obligations to the Public" provide content to this general principle. R1.4 is perhaps the most controversial of the rules of conduct under this first heading. The rule addresses the question of discovery and resignation. If an attorney discovers a plan to engage in fraud, for example, legal ethics obliges the attorney not to abet the wrongdoing and simply to resign. Attorneys have an ethical obligation to remove themselves from the context; usually they have only a negative duty not to participate. R1.4 suggests that HCCPs are held to a different standard, because of the special nature of their implied contract or covenant with society. The commentary to R1.4 states that the obligations of HCCPs to the general public go beyond other professionals inasmuch as HCCPs have a duty actively to prevent organizational misconduct. In short, where other professionals may have a negative duty not to contribute to wrongdoing, HCCPs have a positive duty actively to prevent it. HCCPs should consider resignation only as a last resort, as compliance professionals may be among the only remaining barriers to misconduct. Consequently, they ought not immediately resign if they learn of proposed or ongoing wrongdoing. Rather, the HCCP has a positive duty to "exhaust all internal means available to deter his/her employing organization, its employees or agents from engaging in misconduct." The implication is that HCCPs ought to explore every avenue to prevent misconduct before choosing to resign. This means that an HCCP has an obligation to go to the very highest governing body of a parent organization to report misconduct.

Moreover, R1.4 states: "In the event that resignation becomes necessary, however, the duty to the public takes priority over any duty of confidentiality to the employing organization." An HCCP should report the wrongdoing to public officials "when required by law." In short, the Code states that the implied contract between society and HCCPs obliges HCCPs to blow the whistle if the law requires it. The duty to protect and promote the interests of society, the organization, and patients may in such cases take priority over the duty to protect confidentiality. It is, of course, very important to interpret this section of R1.4 carefully. An HCCP walks a very fine line in such circumstances. He or she must balance a number of competing interests. On the one hand, the HCCP has an obligation to protect the general public. As an employee, however, the HCCP may owe loyalty to the firm. Finally, each HCCP has obligations to the profession. In short, he or she has an obligation to other HCCPs to pursue the good of the profession, or at least not to harm the profession. Naturally, HCCPs can cause the integrity of the profession harm if they themselves become relaters, pursuing profit at the expense of their employers.

The Code attempts to provide guidance to help HCCPs resolve this kind of ethical dilemma by balancing these competing interests. Note that the Code says only that an HCCP should report wrongdoing "when required by law." It does not say that HCCPs should report when they have moral justification to do so. The Code does not recommend that HCCPs aspire to moral heroism. Moral heroes put themselves at personal risk to do what morality permits, but does not require. For example, whistleblowers may commit supererogatory acts when they blow the whistle for moral reasons and at great personal risk, even though there is no moral or legal obligation to do so. Moral heroes go beyond the call of duty—often at their own peril. It is known that whistleblowers fair poorly at the hands of their companies. Most whistleblowers are fired; they are often blackballed by their industries.

Note also that the Code does not even say that an HCCP should blow the whistle when he or she has a moral obligation to do so. In effect, the Code recommends that HCCPs weigh a moral obligation to report against the harm that this would cause the profession. When HCCPs become relaters, this undermines the trust that health administrators place in them. If health administrators do not trust HCCPs, then HCCPs cannot do their jobs. If HCCPs cannot do their jobs, they cannot protect the general public. In short, the Code recommends that HCCPs balance a moral obligation to report against their moral obligations to the general public; they should prioritize the latter over the former. HCCPs should report only when there is a strict legal obligation to do so.

From the relation of HCCPs to the general public, the Code then addresses the relation of HCCPs to employing organizations as next in order of importance. In "Principles II: Obligations to the Employing Organization," HCCPs publicly acclaim their promise to: (1) serve employing organizations with the highest sense of integrity; (2) exercise unprejudiced and unbiased judgment; and (3) promote effective compliance programs.

In ethics, integrity is a technical term with a precise meaning. It is a quality or a state of being complete or undivided. The character of persons with integrity consists of habits of mind and will that incline them to do the right thing for the right reasons. In short, people with integrity have it all. In this section, the Code is explicit about what integrity should mean to HCCPs. HCCPs have a moral obligation to serve their employing organizations in a competent and professional manner. First, HCCPs should have "current and general knowledge of all relevant fields of knowledge that reasonably might be expected of a compliance professional." Second, they should act to the best of their abilities to: (1) ensure that employing organizations comply with the law (R2.2); (2) investigate misconduct with due diligence (R2.3); (3) keep senior management and the highest governing board informed (R2.4); (4) protect from retaliation employees who report misconduct (R2.5); and (5) respect confidentiality (R2.6).

To be able to exercise unprejudiced and unbiased judgment, the Code requires that HCCPs take care to avoid conflict of interest. As suggested above, because a code of ethics should regulate the actual behavior of professionals to be effective, it should not merely list principles and unattainable ideals. It should be specific and honest. A code should thus address those areas that pose as special temptations to members. Conflict of interest is one such area.

There are two kinds of conflict of interest: (1) conflicts between self-interest and the interests of clients; and (2) conflicts that divide loyalties between two or more clients or between a client and a third party. As to the first, the Code requires that HCCPs avoid "actual, potential or perceived conflicts of interest." If an HCCP cannot avoid a conflict of interest, then he or she should disclose the conflict or remove him- or herself from it.[5]

The Code recognizes that HCCPs might find themselves in circumstances similar to the Challenger case, when an employer's wishes will contradict professional ethics. HCCPs need not rely solely on personal beliefs to decide such matters, but now may consult what the Code says about such circumstances. The Code states clearly that HCCPs should not allow loyalty to individuals in the employing organization with whom they have developed a professional or personal relationship to override obligations to society and to their employing organizations. For those who find themselves in Robert Lund's position, R2.7 and its commentary observes that the HCCP is not a neutral party. "Thinking like a compliance professional" may require courageous action that contradicts the wishes of individual managers. The duty to the organization may require such action even if it comes at the expense of close relationships. Thus, the primary duty of the HCCP is to ensure that the organization obeys the law and acts ethically.

Again, as suggested earlier, a code of professional ethics should not be self-serving. Professional associations sometimes use a code of professional ethics to protect the interests of the profession at the expense of the general public or their clients. In "Principle III: Obligations to the Profession," the Code focuses strictly on the relation of ethical standards to compliance tasks. The HCCP ought always to place duty above fear or favor. Integrity, honesty, courage, and fairness are principles that should guide action in the investigation of misconduct. In short, each HCCP has a duty to act in a manner that maintains the integrity and lasting legacy of the profession. It is hoped that this, in turn, will encourage public support for the recognition of health care compliance as a profession.

For example, consistent with R2.6, R3.2 states that HCCPs should protect confidential information about the business affairs of employing organizations. If HCCPs were consistently to breach confidentiality, then this behavior would erode trust in the profession and impair the ability of compliance professionals to obtain such information from others in the future. Failure to obtain information impedes the ability to fulfill obligations to the general public. The commentary to R3.2 also cautions HCCPs to work closely with legal counsel to protect confidentiality in order to prevent the misuse and abuse of the work product of HCCPs in litigation. Finally, to uphold the integrity of the profession, HCCPs also need to be truthful about their own qualifications, not damage the reputation or prospects of other HCCPs, and maintain competence and knowledge about current industry practices and laws (R3.3–5).

CONCLUSION

In the Challenger case, Jerald Mason asked Robert Lund to think like a manager, and not like an engineer. When Lund did so, he failed to follow established guidelines intended to help professionals "think like engineers." How ought a person "think like a compliance professional?" The Code of Ethics for Health Care Compliance Professionals shows the way. First, the Code makes clear that HCCPs share a commitment to an ideal of service to society and the health care industry. Then, the Code sets forth ethical principles on the basis of this ideal. The ethical principles, in turn, ground rules of conduct, which provide HCCPs with concrete ethical standards for the sort of behavior each should expect of one another. The relation of HCCPs to the general public, employing organizations or clients, and the legacy of the profession requires them to uphold the highest standards of professionalism, integrity, and competence.

It is argued in Chapter 1 that professional standards of conduct are born of individual and collective actions. Such standards are not "learned at a mother's knee," but as part of a professional culture developed and sustained by formal professional associations and as part of a larger professional community. HCCA has begun the hard work of professional ethical development with the development and dissemination of a code of ethics for HCCPs, but this is just a beginning.

A code of professional ethics becomes effective only when it is *integrated into the culture of a profession and into the structures of a professional association*. Thus, professional ethical development requires more than just a professional code of conduct, or a set of guidelines and rules. The institutionalization of value commitments across the profession requires the development of a professional ethical culture, the integration of value commitments throughout the structures of a professional association, and the fusion of ethical reflection into the daily practices of all professionals. Responsibility for professional ethical development must extend from national through regional leaders, all the way to front-line practitioners in the field. This goal requires communication with, involvement of, and commitment to professional ethical development at all levels of the profession. How to do this remains one of the difficult challenges that HCCA faces as it matures as an association.

The last point raises an important issue. If a code of professional ethics holds members responsible for the integrity of the profession, it should also hold them accountable. Again, a code of ethics ought to be both policeable and policed. Granted that HCCA does not have the state-enforced power to discipline members legally, the association should make provisions for applying penalties to ensure discipline. Violations should be subject to limited discipline. Expulsion from the professional association is typically the severest penalty, together with public exposure of the act. Censure is a more frequent penalty. If it does not make such provision, then a code is no more than a set of ideals. Although society has yet officially to recognize health care compliance as a profession through state licensure, HCCA should continue to develop the practice of health care compliance as a profession. Unless a professional association demonstrates that it holds its own ranks accountable, then society has no basis for according special privileges to members of the profession. If HCCPs fail to live up to their own ethical guidelines, they should know that they risk, at the very least, censure by the association. The Code represents only partial fulfillment of the association's moral obligations to society to set high standards of conduct for HCCPs. Though HCCA has begun the hard work of professional ethical development with the publication of the Code, much work yet needs be done to hold HCCPs accountable.

NOTES

1. This introductory material also appeared in M.E. Meaney, *An HCCA Code of Ethics for Health Care Compliance Professionals*, 1:3 J. HEALTH CARE COMPLIANCE 42–43 (1999).
2. *See* Chapter 1, *Professional Ethical Development in Health Care Compliance.*
3. *See* Chapter 2, *The Compliance Officer: Delimiting the Domain.*
4. HEALTH CARE COMPLIANCE ASSOCIATION, CODE OF ETHICS FOR HEALTH CARE COMPLIANCE PROFESSIONALS (Nov. 1999).
5. For a more detailed discussion of conflict of interest, *see* Chapter 6, *Conflicts of Interest and Conflicts of Loyalty.*

Conflicts of Interest and Conflicts of Loyalty

Christine Parker

INTRODUCTION

The work of in-house compliance professionals, like other profession-als, is laden with potential for conflict—between the professional's own interests and his or her professional duties, between loyalty to the em-ployer and independent professional judgment, between duties of confi-dentiality to the employer and duties of disclosure to regulators and the public, and between loyalty to individual employees of an entity and duties to the entity as a whole.[1] The multiple roles of most compliance profes-sionals within their organizations make them even more vulnerable to po-tential conflicts of interest and conflicts of loyalty than other professionals. In a survey of occupational stress among health care compliance officers, Heller and Guetter have concluded that compliance officers are more likely than most other professional groups to experience stress associated with role conflict, as well as workload and role ambiguity.[2] Because of the rapid growth in compliance program implementation in some industries, including health care, the role of the compliance professional is not always well defined. Compliance may often be only one part of somebody's job, especially in smaller organizations, or where the compliance program is very new. This can lead to confusion and to conflicts between the compli-ance responsibility and other key management responsibilities. Even within the compliance role itself, the compliance professional's simulta-

I would like to thank Simson Chu for diligent research assistance, and Joseph E. Murphy and Jan C. Heller for helpful comments on a draft of this chapter.

neous responsibility for consulting, managing, and policing[3] can often exacerbate or create conflicts of interest and conflicts of loyalty.

This chapter discusses how to identify and respond, first, to conflicts of interest, and second, to conflicts of loyalty. A *conflict of interest* occurs where some personal or financial interest of the compliance professional (this is taken to include interests of the compliance professional's relatives or associates) has a tendency to influence the professional's judgment on his or her employer's behalf. Conflicts of interest threaten to compromise the professional's duties of loyalty, diligence, confidentiality, and care to the interests of the employer. A *conflict of loyalty* occurs where the compliance professional's duty of loyalty to his or her employer, especially the duty of confidentiality, conflicts with his or her duties to external values and entities, including duties to obey the law, to uphold the values of the compliance profession, and to protect public health and safety. A compliance professional may also face an internal conflict of loyalty between loyalty to the organization as a whole and its compliance program, and loyalty to an individual officer within the organization, such as a particular chief executive officer (CEO) to whom the compliance officer reports.

An effective professional can distinguish between the different types of conflict, and knows how to identify and resolve conflicts that can give rise to legal or ethical problems. The most effective professionals will also minimize problems with both conflicts of interest and conflicts of loyalty through appropriate design of the compliance work role, and reporting and decision-making structures. The final section of this chapter outlines some practical suggestions for how to design the role of the compliance professional, and the compliance program, to avoid or resolve conflicts of interest and conflicts of loyalty before they become a problem.

IDENTIFYING CONFLICTS OF INTEREST

A *conflict of interest* occurs where some personal or financial interest of the compliance professional has a tendency to influence his or her professional judgment on the employer's behalf.[4] Compliance officers are hired to exercise independent professional judgment in advising and assisting the employing organization to implement a compliance program, to monitor compliance, and to engage in corrective action where wrongdoing is found or suspected. A conflict of interest is a betrayal of trust. The employer trusts the compliance professional to act and advise in its best interests. A conflict of interest means that some other factor affects the professional's judgment or actions. A good test for conflicts of interests is the "trust test": "Would others [employer, clients, colleagues] trust my judgment if they knew I was in this situation?"[5]

All employees have other roles and interests in addition to their employee role that may affect their judgment in carrying out their employee or professional duties; for example, an interest in getting home early to spend time with family and friends, or an interest in putting a good "spin" on the performance of one's role in order to keep a job or get a pay raise or promotion.[6] All professionals need to be honest with themselves about what extraneous factors may affect their judgment in particular situations. Ethical and legal problems with conflicts of interest arise where the professional has some interest or association beyond and above the usual, everyday factors that might affect that professional's judgment. Conflicts of interest compromise the professional's duties of loyalty, diligence, confidentiality, and care to the interests of the employer. As the U.S. Health Care Compliance Association's (HCCA) Code of Ethics for Health Care Compliance Professionals[7] puts it, "Health care compliance professionals should serve their employing organizations with the highest sense of integrity, should exercise unprejudiced and unbiased judgment on their behalf, and should promote effective compliance programs."

Compliance professionals will potentially encounter conflicts of interest arising from many of the same situations and temptations that other professionals face. These include where the compliance professional has a business association, a direct or indirect financial interest, or other substantial interest, including in relation to a family member or friend (or perhaps even an enemy), that could affect his or her judgment in carrying out his or her responsibilities. Some of the "classic" situations of conflict of interest, and examples of how they might apply to compliance professionals, include the following:

- *Self-dealing*: For example, a compliance professional uses his or her position to influence a contracting decision to give work to a firm in which the compliance professional is involved; or influences the organization to enter into a contract to buy or sell property with the compliance professional's friend or associate.
- *Accepting benefits/bribery*: For example, a compliance professional receives a kickback from providing compliance consulting or inde-

pendent auditing work to a particular firm; or receives a gift for buying computer software from a particular supplier.

*   *Using the employer's property for private advantage*: For example, a compliance professional uses the employer's photocopier to copy leaflets advertising his or her spouse's business.
*   *Using the employer's confidential information to personal advantage*: Many compliance professionals have access to extensive confidential information about the employer's business, financial performance, and internal scandals and breaches, that may be abused. For example, a compliance professional sells shares in the company, or advises a close friend to sell shares in the company after learning about an impending major regulatory investigation that is likely to lead to a negative market reaction when it becomes public (insider trading); the compliance professional sells the story of a compliance scandal in the organization to a muckraking magazine or talk show; or the compliance professional leaks information about a new product line to a competitor, before it becomes public.

In addition to these conflicts of interest, situations in which a conflict of interest might affect the professional judgment of a compliance professional in particular include:

*   *Investigations*: Where the compliance professional must investigate the integrity and compliance record of a relative, friend, or enemy in relation to a suspected compliance breach, or where a relative, friend, or enemy is a candidate for employment and due diligence requires a compliance check.
*   *Job incentives*: Where the compliance professional's job incentives are tied to annual sales, this means that the compliance professional's interest in the short-term profits of the organization may conflict with the duty to ensure compliance with the law. It might be better to tie the compliance professional's incentives to long-term stock performance.

Compliance professionals will also be especially vulnerable to a unique set of conflicts of interest that arise from the multiple, and potentially conflicting, roles that compliance professionals often have within an organization. Of course, compliance professionals need not hold conflicting roles in order to encounter problematic conflicts of interest; nevertheless, most will need to be especially vigilant to avoid conflicts of interest arising from conflicts of roles. Conflicts of interest may arise from conflict of roles where either one person simultaneously holds a compliance role and a non-compliance role or where the kaleidoscope of roles included in the job of compliance professional come into conflict.

In the first situation, the person who is the designated compliance officer holds dual roles within the organization. He or she is the designated compliance officer and also holds other key management responsibilities; for example, human resources manager *and* compliance manager, or chief financial officer *and* compliance manager, or general counsel *and* compliance officer. Dual roles are very common at all sorts of organizations. Limited available financial resources or appropriate expertise may make such joint responsibility a practical necessity in particular organizations, especially in small or rural organizations. The joint roles do not, on their face, involve a conflict of interest. But holding both roles does make it more likely that a conflict of interest might arise. (The risk of conflict of interest may, however, be acceptable because it is outweighed by the need to give the compliance officer another senior role in order to ensure his or her "clout" or effectiveness in the organization.)

A compliance professional who holds another managerial position in an organization will have to be vigilant in guarding against conflicts of interest. A conflict of interest may arise where the compliance professional has to make a decision in one role that might have an adverse effect on his or her key area of responsibility in the other role. For example, a Head of Marketing who is also Compliance Officer might need to decide whether to run an advertisement tomorrow, when legal advice suggests it might be misleading, or whether to delay the advertising campaign and lose the competitive advantage. Or, a Compliance Officer who is also Vice President for Human Resources in a trading bank may have to decide whether to terminate the employment of the firm's top sales agent because of failure to disclose certain required product information to customers.

A conflict of interest might also arise from dual roles in the organization where the person in his or her capacity as compliance officer must investigate a potential wrongdoing/mistake in which he or she was directly or indirectly involved personally or as a supervisor in his or her other capacity.[8] For example, a Chief Financial Officer who is also Compliance Officer for a health care provider might discount certain overpayments identified to improve the company's bottom line profits, and then be asked to conduct an investigation into alleged breaches associated with the discounted overpayments. Or, a Nursing Care Director who is also the Compliance Officer in a hospital might need to investigate alleged breaches of quality of care provisions by nurses under his or her supervision who say they were acting according to his or her instructions.

In the second situation, conflicts of interest might arise simply because compliance professionals perform a number of different roles as compliance professionals—including consultant, manager, and investigator.[9] Although these different compliance roles should usually complement each other, at certain times the performance of different roles within the one job may create conflicts of interest for even the most conscientious of compliance professionals. These conflicts are most likely to arise where the compliance professional's *policing* role involves investigating a suspected breach where the compliance professional in his or her *consulting* or training role had previously advised the person under investigation on how to comply. Indeed the compliance role often involves working closely with managers and employees during compliance consulting or training. This may easily give rise to conflicts if the compliance professional later has to investigate the same people with whom he or she has collaborated and become friends. For this reason, it is better, if possible, to keep the investigative role in compliance separate from the consulting and managing roles by employing different staff to carry out the two roles, or hiring independent auditors to conduct serious investigations (this is discussed further in the next section). Conflicts of interest arising from role conflicts may also give rise to conflicts of loyalty (this is discussed further below).

RESPONDING TO CONFLICTS OF INTEREST

Most professionals, including compliance professionals, will find themselves in a potential conflict of interest situation at some stage in their careers. What should a compliance professional do in the face of a possible conflict? It has been observed that having a conflict of interest is not wrong in itself: "To have a conflict of interest is to have a moral problem. What will be morally right or wrong, or at least morally good or bad, is how one resolves that problem."[10] It is not the fact that a conflict of interest arises, but how the compliance professional handles it that will be the critical issue. There are two ways in which a conflict of interest can be handled properly: (1) by avoiding or removing the conflict, or (2) by fully disclosing the conflict to the employer and obtaining the employer's informed consent to continue, despite the conflict. As the HCCA Code of Ethics puts it, compliance professionals "shall take care to avoid any actual, potential or perceived conflicts of interest; to disclose them when they cannot be avoided; and to remove them where possible."[11]

Generally, situations in which a compliance professional's direct personal financial interest conflicts with the duty to the employer should be eliminated, if at all possible. Many such conflicts can and should be avoided in the first place, including self-dealing, abuse of confidential information, and the use of the employer's property for personal financial gain. If a compliance professional does find him- or herself in a situation where he or she has any business association, direct or indirect financial interest, or other interest that could be substantial enough to influence, or appear to influence, his or her judgment, the compliance professional should fully disclose the nature of the business association, financial interest, or other interest to the employing organization.[12] It is not enough to disclose merely that there is a conflict of interest; the details of the conflict must be explained. It will be up to the employer to decide whether the compliance professional should eliminate the conflict of interest, whether the compliance professional will be able to continue as normal, or whether he or she should work under special conditions that minimize or avoid the effects of the conflict of interest, such as absenting him- or herself from certain roles or decision-making processes.

In the special situation in which compliance professionals must investigate a suspected breach where they may have been involved in some way in the conduct being investigated, it is especially important that the compliance professional fully disclose the potential conflict to his or her employer. It is in the performance of investigations that employers rely most heavily on compliance professionals to exercise independent judgment. In particular, the employer relies on the compliance professional to report accurately and truthfully so as not to leave the employing organization vulnerable to any claim, by either regulators or employees, that the investigation was unfair, misleading, or improper. An investigation or report into alleged misconduct that is biased by conflict of interest may not only mislead the employing organization as to the true extent of a noncompliance problem, but also leave the way open for employees to state a claim for wrongful discharge (or denial of due process in jurisdictions where it is recognized), and for government regulators to question the seriousness and intent of the compliance program. The HCCA Code of Ethics gives very helpful guidance as to what is required in this situation:

> If a report, investigation or inquiry into misconduct relates directly or indirectly to activity in which the HCCP [health care compliance professional] was involved in any manner, the HCCP must disclose in writing the precise nature of that involvement to the senior management of the employing organization before responding to a report or beginning an investigation or inquiry into such matter. Despite this requirement, such involvement in a matter subject to a report, investigation or inquiry will not necessarily prejudice the member's ability to fulfill his/her responsibilities in that regard.[13]

It is wise for a compliance professional to disclose any conflict of interest in writing to the employing organization. But it is particularly important that the exact nature of a conflict of interest in something as serious as an investigation be disclosed in writing to the employer. This is both to ensure that the employer is fully aware of any bias that may exist in the investigation process and report, and to protect the compliance professional against any claims that he or she tried to cover up the conflict of interest.

IDENTIFYING CONFLICTS OF LOYALTY

Conflicts of *interest* arise where it is clear that the compliance professional's primary duty is owed to the employer, yet some direct or indirect personal or financial interest of the compliance professional threatens to interfere with that overriding duty of care, loyalty, confidentiality, and diligence to the employer. The duty to the employer must prevail either through elimination of the conflict, or through disclosure and obtaining consent to continue. Conflicts of *loyalty* are more complicated. Where there is a conflict of loyalty, the duty to the employer conflicts (or at least appears to conflict) with some other valid professional duty, and it is unclear which should prevail. For example, in Heller and Guetter's survey, compliance officers reported that conflict between "the government's and the board's expectations and the way business just gets done," being expected "to ensure compliance with the deals and contracts that some senior management made and signed without input or review by the compliance officer," and feeling responsible for compliance problems they uncovered but could not resolve put them in very uncomfortable positions.[14] Here the compliance professionals experience conflict between loyalty to senior management's idea of normal business practice and their professional responsibilities owed to the organization as whole.

There are two main categories of conflict of loyalties that can arise for a compliance professional: (1) where a loyalty to an individual within the organization conflicts with the duty of loyalty owed to the organization as a whole, and (2) where the compliance professional's duties to the law, his or her profession, or to the public conflicts with the duty owed to the employing organization. For a compliance professional, a conflict of loyalty will often revolve around the issue of whether to breach the duty of confidentiality owed to one party (either the employer or, perhaps, an individual within the organization) in order to fulfill the duty owed to the other.

The first situation, where a loyalty to an individual within the organization conflicts with the duty of loyalty owed to the organization as a whole, is really a situation of *divided* loyalties, rather than *conflicted* loyalties. Such divided loyalties can easily develop from the earlier-described conflict of interest situations. The multiple, and sometimes conflicting, roles of the compliance professional mean that compliance professionals will often develop loyalties to individual officers and employees of the organization. These might potentially conflict with the primary loyalty owed to the organization as a whole to exercise independent professional judgment in advising and assisting the employing organization to implement a compliance program, to monitor compliance, and to engage in corrective action where wrongdoing is found or suspected. At any given time any constituent individual or unit of the organization—whether CEO, business unit, or unit head, or employee with whom the compliance professional is communicating—could have interests at odds with those of the corporation as a whole. Situations in which divided loyalties might arise include:

- where it is unclear to whom within the organization the compliance professional reports and is ultimately responsible, and where different managers within the organization have conflicting instructions or views on what the compliance professional should do
- where the compliance professional reports to a business unit head, the general counsel, or the chief financial officer, and this person is instructing the compliance professional to do something that is not in

the interests of the compliance of the entity as a whole according to the compliance professional's professional judgment
- where the compliance professional discovers some information about an individual employee's possible breach and the employee wants the compliance professional to give him or her confidential information on how to respond or protect him- or herself from repercussions, or where an individual employee or officer wants to communicate in confidence with the compliance professional about potentially illegal behavior

The principle that applies to resolve issues in the first situation of divided loyalties among internal constituencies is relatively simple. Generally, the overriding duty is owed to the employing organization as a whole entity, not to any individual officer, employee, or business unit. For example, the HCCA Code of Ethics provides that:

> Conflicts of interest can also create divided loyalties. HCCPs shall not permit loyalty to individuals in the employing organization with whom they have developed a professional or a personal relationship to interfere with or supersede the duty of loyalty to the employing organization and/or the superior responsibility of upholding the law, ethical business conduct and this Code of Ethics.[15]

In practice it may sometimes be difficult to identify who in the organization represents the entity as a whole for the purposes of the compliance professional. Ultimately, it is the board of directors or highest governing authority that generally represents the organization as a whole. Individual employees should be informed that the compliance professional has a duty to exercise professional judgment in the interests of the effective implementation and operation of the compliance program of the organization as a whole, not according to the instructions of any individual; moreover, the compliance professional must not allow any loyalty to any individual in the organization to interfere with the compliance function. If necessary, conflicting instructions must be reported to the board level and resolved there. As discussed below, divided loyalties can be avoided to some extent by ensuring that the compliance officer and compliance unit report directly to the CEO and, preferably, also to the board or board compliance or audit committee.

In the second situation a true *conflict of loyalty* exists. The compliance professional's duties to the law, the profession, or to the public conflict with the duty owed to the employer. A problem of divided loyalties may exacerbate this sort of conflict of loyalties. For example, an environmental compliance officer reports to the general manager of a factory site. The general manager is cutting the budget so that the compliance officer does not have sufficient resources to remove some old toxic waste in barrels on the site. The CEO at the head office wants environmental compliance taken seriously, but has devolved budget responsibility to the general managers of the sites, in addition to the devolved compliance reporting structure. To whom is the compliance officer's duty owed—to the general manager on-site, or to the CEO and the compliance officer's own independent professional judgment that the barrels ought to be removed because of the likelihood that local groundwater will be contaminated or workers exposed to dangerous chemicals?

The very appointment of a compliance professional to help an organization comply with a particular area of regulation creates a potential conflict between a general right (or duty) to prevent and report illegal conduct, and the duty of loyalty and confidentiality to the employing organization. At the U.S. Practicing Law Institute's 1999 corporate compliance conference, one presenter highlighted the conflicts faced by compliance staff by entitling his presentation, "Some Organizations Call It 'Compliance Officer'—Some Call It 'Designated Felon.'" The presenter commented on the "critical conflict" between the compliance professional's

> . . . duty of loyalty to the organization, and his/her right to disclose wrongdoing to responsible regulatory authorities. . . . [T]he conflict is triggered if and when a formal compliance finding or recommendation is made in respect to the incident, and is willfully ignored by the organization, placing the team member's accountabilities and responsibilities at odds with the decision maker's.[16]

Where there is a conflict of loyalty, the ethical and legal problem will often revolve around whether the compliance professional should disclose confidential information that he or she has discovered in the course of his or her employment, where that information may need to be disclosed in the public interest or according to regulatory rules. Although the general rule is that compliance professionals, like other professionals, should not disclose an employer's confidential information, professional ethics and the duty to the public demand that "under certain circumstances confidentiality must yield to other values or concerns, for example, to stop an act which creates appreciable risk to health and safety, or to reveal a confidence when necessary to comply with a subpoena or other legal process."[17] The dilemma will arise where the compliance professional has identified a compliance problem, but relevant officers in the organization will not authorize the action required to address the problem; or, where the interpretation differs between the organization and the government as to what action compliance requires, and the compliance professional's judgment is that the government's view should be followed.

Consider the following examples of situations in which compliance professionals may feel that they should blow the whistle on noncompliance:

- U.S. federal law makes it unlawful to retain possession of known overpayments associated with forms of misconduct when the overpayments are received under a federal health care program.[18] A compliance professional in a health care provider organization has conducted an audit and discovered various probable overpayments. The compliance professional believes that the overpayments should be disclosed. But the general counsel's opinion is that it is arguable whether some of the payments are overpayments and the CEO proposes to follow the general counsel's advice and not disclose. The board of directors agrees with the CEO. The compliance professional strongly suspects that the CEO has instructed the general counsel to come up with any conceivable argument that might support nondisclosure, regardless of how likely it is to be accepted.
- The same situation as above except that the compliance officer does not believe that the disclosure of overpayments is required by the law, but that disclosure would be highly desirable under the Department of Health and Human Services (HHS) Office of Inspector General's (OIG) self-disclosure protocol.[19] The CEO thinks that it is not appropriate to disclose all the overpayments immediately and wants to wait three months before making any disclosure. The compliance officer believes that in three months the HHS OIG will not consider the disclosure timely enough to give the company the benefits of voluntary self-disclosure.
- A compliance officer in a nursing home company receives reports that the quality of care standards are routinely ignored in one of the

company's remote nursing homes. The compliance officer wants to conduct an investigation, but the chief financial officer says that the company does not have the money at the moment to send the compliance officer to the site of this nursing home or to hire an independent consultant to conduct an investigation; further, the compliance officer is needed in the head office to coordinate monitoring of health care fraud compliance because the company is currently under investigation by the HHS OIG.

* A compliance officer in a nursing home company conducts an investigation and discovers that a remote nursing home routinely ignores quality of care standards that put residents' health, and sometimes lives, at risk. The CEO says that the nursing home is financially marginal anyway, and has therefore decided that the home will not take any new residents. Operations will be wound down so that the home can be closed in about three years' time. The compliance officer believes that either compliance should be improved or the nursing home closed down immediately.

These situations raise true conflicts of loyalty because, if the compliance professional acts according to what he or she believes to be professional duty by disclosing the employing organization's noncompliance,[20] then the employing organization may dismiss him or her for breach of the duty of loyalty to the employer.[21]

On the other hand, if the compliance professional does nothing, then he or she has failed in his or her professional duty by leaving the employer open to the possibility of civil or criminal prosecution for noncompliance. The compliance professional could also lose his or her professional reputation and even his or her job if the compliance breach becomes known to regulators or the public later. In some cases, professional advisors have also been indicted for aiding and abetting their employer's noncompliance where they have been "over-loyal" to the employer.[22]

RESPONDING TO CONFLICTS OF LOYALTY

It is advisable for each compliance professional to have a predetermined stance on what he or she would do when faced with a conflict of loyalties (and better still, to spell it out in a written agreement with the employer, as discussed further below). The heat of the moment may make it difficult to judge effectively. Many professionals (including corporate attorneys, as an ethical obligation)[23] find it helpful to follow a process of reporting any potential conflicts of loyalty up the chain to the supreme governing body, and disclosing confidential information externally only if the conflict remains *and* public health and safety are at risk. This is the approach taken by the HCCA Code of Ethics in this respect. It sets out the following "obligations to the public":

R1.1 HCCPs shall not aid, abet or participate in misconduct.

R1.2 HCCPs shall take such steps as are necessary to prevent misconduct by their employing organizations.

R1.3 HCCPs shall cooperate with all official and legitimate government investigations of or inquiries concerning their employing organization.

R1.4 If, in the course of their work, HCCPs become aware of any decision by their employing organization which, if implemented, would constitute misconduct and which will adversely affect the health of patients, residents or clients, the professional shall: (a) refuse to consent to the decision; (b) escalate to the highest governing authority, as appropriate; (c) if serious issues remain unresolved, consider resignation; and (d) report the decision to public officials when required by law.[24]

Further guidance is offered in the following commentary to R1.4:

The duty of a compliance professional goes beyond other professionals in an organizational context, inasmuch as his/her duty to the public includes prevention of organizational misconduct. The compliance professional should exhaust all internal means available to deter his/her employing organization, its employees and agents from engaging in misconduct. HCCPs should consider resignation only as a last resort, since compliance professionals may be the only remaining barrier to misconduct. In the event that resignation becomes necessary, however, the duty to the public takes priority over any duty of confidentiality to the employing organization. A letter of resignation should set forth to senior management and the highest governing body of the employing organization the precise conditions that necessitate his/her action. In complex organizations, the highest governing body may be the highest governing body of a parent corporation.

This implies that, in the earlier scenarios, it is only the last situation in which it is clear that the compliance professional could be entitled to report the noncompliance to a regulator, because patient health is at risk. In the first situation, the compliance professional will need to decide whether he or she is at risk of personal liability for aiding and abetting the concealment of the overpayments. If so, then the compliance professional should consider whether the situation is serious enough to warrant resigning, with a letter to the board of directors setting out the circumstances. In the second and third situations, the compliance professional needs to escalate the situation to the board of directors for a decision. Neither situation is likely to justify resignation or public disclosure. Public disclosure would be appropriate only if the noncompliance remains unaddressed and public health or safety is at risk.

In some situations where a compliance professional faces a very serious conflict of loyalties, the best option may be to resign and seek a more congenial job with an employer with a better attitude toward compliance. Indeed, compliance professionals live with the constant tension of a dual role. The organization hired the compliance professional to exercise independent judgment in implementing and operating the compliance program, but the organization also demands loyalty from the compliance professional, including nondisclosure of confidential information (including breaches) and no action that might harm the interests of the organization (such as reporting noncompliance to the appropriate authority or even perhaps insisting on implementing measures that would ensure compliance but that might harm other business objectives). When these two roles of compliance professionals come into conflict, they face the dilemma of whether to resign (on principle), be dismissed (if unscrupulous management wants to rid the company of a principled compliance manager), or face the constant potential of regulatory action against the organization for corporate noncompliance and even prosecution against the compliance professional him- or herself.

DESIGN THE COMPLIANCE PROGRAM TO AVOID CONFLICTS OF INTEREST AND CONFLICTS OF LOYALTY

Many of the unique conflicts of interest and conflicts of loyalty that compliance professionals face arise from either lack of clarity about their responsibilities or conflict in their roles. Many conflicts of interest and conflicts of loyalty could therefore be avoided, or at least more speedily resolved, through appropriate design of the compliance program and the compliance professional's job description to avoid conflicts of roles where possible, to allow the compliance professional to take conflicts directly to the board, and to clarify the compliance professional's duty to exercise *independent* professional judgment. Moreover, it is crucial that compliance professionals wield "clout." Just as various conventions have grown up to protect the independence of auditors and general counsel, so should the place of compliance professionals within organizations be protected. This section sets out principles of compliance design and practice that can help compliance professionals maintain their professional integrity, buttressed by internal structures that protect independence.

The compliance professional should, if possible, avoid holding competing roles. If possible, the compliance professional should avoid holding other, competing management roles within the organization. In addition, the compliance office should be maintained as a separate unit within the organization. This will reduce conflicts of interest arising from conflicting roles, and also will help avoid conflicts of loyalty arising from the need to exercise independent judgment on compliance issues and other management priorities. For example, the HHS OIG suggests that:

> [T]here is some risk to establishing an independent compliance function if that function is subordinate to the [organization's] general counsel, or comptroller or similar . . . financial officer. Freestanding compliance functions help to ensure independent and objective legal reviews and financial analyses of the institution's compliance efforts and activities. By separating the compliance function from the key management position of general counsel or chief . . . financial officer (where the size and structure of the [organization] make this a feasible option), a system of checks and balances is established to more effectively achieve the goals of the compliance program.[25]

Some organizations may decide that it is better to maintain dual management and compliance functions for a senior officer in order to avoid loss of clout and isolation in the compliance function. If so, it is generally preferable to combine the compliance function with a role, such as general counsel, that also has a tradition of independence and clout. If it is unavoidable that the compliance officer also holds some other key operational management function within a small organization, then the compliance responsibility should be assigned to a well-respected manager with a record of sensitivity to potential conflicts.

Ideally, to avoid conflicts of interest in investigations, designated attorneys from the in-house legal team (or members of internal audit) might conduct audits and investigations. The organization would use compliance staff for consulting functions only, together with different in-house attorneys, if the organization is large enough. Alternatively, different compliance staff could be involved in investigations than in consulting and training. This could mean that the organization hires a permanent team of compliance professionals, some of whom specialize in consulting, training, and compliance management and others in investigations and audits. For many organizations, maintaining this level of permanent staff will be unrealistic. A further alternative might be to hire external investigators or auditors on special occasions as required to conduct investigations of serious suspected breaches and periodic thorough compliance audits, while using permanent compliance or legal staff to conduct routine audits and investigations, as well as to provide consulting services.

The compliance professional should be subject to appropriate reporting structures that provide checks and balances in the compliance structure. The professional integrity and independence of compliance professionals can be buttressed by appropriate reporting structures and by checks and balances in the corporate governance structure. Compliance professionals should always report directly to the CEO rather than to business unit heads or other key managers (such as the general counsel or chief financial officer), and should have a dotted line reporting relationship directly to a board audit, compliance, or social responsibility committee and to the board of directors itself.[26] This structure will avoid many potential conflicts of loyalty where business objectives of a line manager conflict with compliance responsibilities. It also allows the compliance professional to escalate unresolved conflicts quickly to a level in the company where they can be authoritatively resolved. For example, if there are competing messages about compliance and profit-making or production goals being sent down the line from on high, then the compliance professional has the authority to ask top managers to resolve the conflict. If a compliance problem is a matter of an individual doing the wrong thing against company policy, then this reporting structure would provide the compliance professional with the clout to ensure that the individual is quickly held accountable by higher management.

Where it is considered unavoidable (or desirable) that the compliance officer holds another management responsibility in addition to the compliance role, appropriate reporting structures can help this person to avoid conflicts of interest. For example, the compliance officer could report to a strong and active compliance steering committee, as well as to the CEO and board. The steering committee would meet regularly to set compliance priorities and take responsibility for resolving conflicts between the compliance officer's competing responsibilities. A compliance steering committee made up of well-respected and high-level people from throughout the organization can command the independence and respect that an individual compliance officer, who also holds other management responsibilities, will lack in some situations.

It is particularly important to determine the reporting lines and responsibilities in relation to any compliance investigations before they begin in order to avoid later conflicts. When setting out the scope and method of any compliance investigation or audit, the organization, compliance officer, and any external investigative team should determine to whom the investigative team will be accountable. This choice will have implications for the credibility, independence, and effectiveness of the internal investigation. The degree of independence and credibility may in turn impact the level of cooperation and credibility that the organization may have with government entities investigating potential violations. Ideally, the audit or investigative team should report to a separate committee of an organization's board of directors and to the chief compliance officer.[27]

The compliance professionals should, if possible, have an employment agreement that sets out clear role expectations and protections for his or her independent professional judgment. Clarifying the role and responsibilities of the compliance professional can be an important way of avoiding conflict, and also setting out clearly how the compliance professional should resolve conflicts that do occur. One way of clarifying role expectations and responsibilities between the compliance professional and the employer is by means of an employment agreement. At the least, every compliance professional should try to obtain an agreement, or at least a job description, that sets out the scope and function of the position and its responsibilities so that the compliance professional does not have to spend time arguing about it later, especially when a conflict arises between compliance and other management priorities. The employment agreement should set out the standards for conduct of the compliance professional, and also make it clear that the compliance professional owes duties both to the employer *and* to the law and the profession, that the compliance role is one of *independent* professional judgment. It should also set out agreed procedures both for the organization to remove the compliance professional (so that he or she cannot be fired at will) and for the compliance professional to disclose noncompliance to the highest governing authority of the organization. It should also set out procedures to follow if the compliance professional finds him- or herself in a situation of conflict of interest or conflict of loyalty (for example, a procedure of reporting conflicts of loyalty up the chain to the board of directors, and then resigning or disclosing if public health and safety is at risk, as discussed earlier). At the very least this should alert the employer to the dual responsibilities of the compliance professional, as an independent professional and as an employee.[28]

Ideally, an employment agreement would also protect the independence and clout of the compliance professional.[29] For example, in some organizations, the chief compliance officer shares the same protection in employment as the chief financial officer; the compliance officer cannot be terminated or even resign voluntarily without the matter going to a meeting of the board so that the directors can satisfy themselves that the termination or resignation is not occurring for the wrong reasons. The employment agreement might also be used to ensure that the compliance professional is guaranteed the necessary resources and support to get the job done.

The compliance professional should maintain involvement in a professional network of other compliance professionals outside the organization. Finally, compliance professionals should aim to maintain contact and involvement with a network of other compliance professionals through informal friendship and involvement in professional associations and meetings. There are two reasons for this. First, participating in the professional community will give the compliance professional opportunities to become aware of and discuss up-to-date ethical and professional issues, including conflicts. It will provide a constant source of support, advice, and expertise on issues to watch for, techniques to become more effective, and wisdom in how to handle difficult situations.[30] It will remind the compliance professional of the standards that he or she is expected to live up to and give him or her support in doing so.

Second, the dual loyalties of the compliance professional will sometimes make compliance employment precarious. Although compliance professionals may have some protection from wrongful discharge, being an active part of a professional network will make it much easier to find a new job if the compliance professional has to resign or is laid off. Indeed, it should be an important function of professional associations to support professional integrity and independence by giving concrete support to professionals employed by organizations who risk their livelihoods by standing up for values to which they are committed.[31] For example, if a company undermines or terminates a compliance officer for advocating that money be spent on improving quality of care standards in a hospital, the professional association could issue press releases about what has happened and offer financial support to the professional who has lost his or her job. More realistically, the existence of the professional network also provides a network of potential alternative job opportunities for compliance professionals unhappy with the support offered in their current jobs, or facing dismissal as the price of their integrity.

CONCLUSION

Compliance professionals have a high probability of facing a potential conflict of interest or conflict of loyalty. In both cases, however, there are a few simple things that the compliance professional can do to prepare him- or herself so that the potential conflict of interest or conflict of loyalty does not lead to illegal, unethical, or unwise behavior. It is how the professional handles the conflict, not the fact that the conflict arises, that is the crucial thing. Organizations hire professionals because they are expected to act diligently and independently in very complex situations. There is nothing more complex and delicate than compliance management, so it is wise to be prepared.

A number of potential conflicts of interest can be "designed out" of the compliance professional's role from the beginning by not giving compliance professionals competing roles, if possible; by making sure that the compliance professional is part of an appropriate reporting structure; and by setting out mutual expectations clearly in an employment agreement. Certain other conflicts of interest can and should be completely avoided (such as self-dealing, abuse of confidential information, and use of the employer's property for personal gain), while some can be handled by disclosing the conflict to the employer and receiving permission to continue to act. Conflicts of loyalty, on the other hand, can pose the most difficult dilemmas for compliance (and other) professionals. It is here that a compliance professional will occasionally have to choose whether to "blow the whistle" to the board on a colleague or superior with whom he or she has worked closely or to conclude that an issue is important enough to resign or even report to a regulator. In making these judgment calls, compliance professionals will need all the support and advice they can get from the community of compliance colleagues in their industry. The HCCA's Code of Ethics is one place where some of that wisdom is distilled into guidance for action. But nothing replaces sharing experiences and war stories with other professionals as a means of learning how to practice ethical behavior in very difficult commercial situations.

NOTES

1. There also can be potential conflicts of interest for outside professionals including conflicts in representing different clients. These types of conflicts are not discussed here.
2. J.C. Heller & J.R. Guetter, *Is Compliance Officer a Tough Job, or What?*, 1:3 J. HEALTH CARE COMPLIANCE 45–50 (1999).
3. For an in-depth discussion of these roles, see Chapter 3, *A Model for the Compliance Professional: Consulting, Policing, and Managing.*
4. In general, a professional will also be taken to have a personal or financial interest in a matter, for the purposes of conflict-of-interest rules, if a relative or business associate has an interest in the matter.
5. M. McDonald, *Ethics and Conflict of Interest*, available on the Internet at <http://www.ethics.ubc.ca/mcdonald/conflict.html>.
6. Rule 2.8 of the Health Care Compliance Association's Code of Ethics for Health Care Compliance Professionals states that HCCPs shall not mislead employing organizations about the results that can be achieved through the use of their services. HEALTH CARE COMPLIANCE ASSOCIATION, CODE OF ETHICS FOR HEALTH CARE COMPLIANCE PROFESSIONALS, Rule 2.8 PROFESSIONALS (1999).
7. The HCCA is one of the first associations to set out a code of ethics to help guide compliance professionals. It contains very helpful advice and guidance for all compliance professionals, not just health care compliance professionals.
8. As is discussed below, this conflict can also arise even for compliance officers who do not hold any other organizational functions.
9. *See* Chapter 3, *A Model for the Compliance Professional: Consulting, Policing, and Managing.*
10. M. Davis, *Conflict of Interest, in* 1 ENCYCLOPEDIA OF APPLIED ETHICS 589–95 (R. Chadwick ed., 1998).
11. HEALTH CARE COMPLIANCE ASSOCIATION, CODE OF ETHICS FOR HEALTH CARE COMPLIANCE PROFESSIONALS, Rule 2.7 (1999).
12. *See* HEALTH CARE COMPLIANCE ASSOCIATION, CODE OF ETHICS FOR HEALTH CARE COMPLIANCE PROFESSIONALS, Commentary to Rule 2.7 (1999).
13. HEALTH CARE COMPLIANCE ASSOCIATION, CODE OF ETHICS FOR HEALTH CARE COMPLIANCE PROFESSIONALS, Commentary to Rule 2.7 (1999).
14. J.C. Heller & J.R. Guetter, *Is Compliance Officer a Tough Job, or What?*, 1:3 J. HEALTH CARE COMPLIANCE 45–50 (1999).
15. HEALTH CARE COMPLIANCE ASSOCIATION, CODE OF ETHICS FOR HEALTH CARE COMPLIANCE PROFESSIONALS, Rule 2.7 (1999).
16. H. Zinn, *Some Organizations Call It "Compliance Officer"—Some Call It "Designated Felon": Considerations in Designating, Empowering, and Supporting Your Organization's Compliance Leader*, 1 CORP. COMPLIANCE 533–47 (1999 PLI).

17. From HEALTH CARE COMPLIANCE ASSOCIATION, CODE OF ETHICS FOR HEALTH CARE COMPLIANCE PROFESSIONALS, Rule 2.6 (1999).

18. G. Imperato, *Internal Investigations, Government Investigations, Whistleblower Concerns: Techniques to Protect Your Health Care Organization*, 51 ALA. L. REV. 205–38 (1999).

19. *See* Department of Health and Human Services, Office of Inspector General, Provider Self-Disclosure Protocol, 63 Fed. Reg. 58.399 (Oct. 30, 1998).

20. The compliance officer could even conceivably run a *qui tam* lawsuit under the False Claims Act in relation to noncompliance associated with fraudulent health care payments. *See* G. Imperato, *Internal Investigations, Government Investigations, Whistleblower Concerns: Techniques to Protect Your Health Care Organization*, 51 ALA. L. REV. 205–38 (1999).

21. However, in many states, courts recognize a public policy exception to employment-at-will so that employees who are fired for refusing to violate the law can recover damages for wrongful discharge. *See* E. Chambliss, *Title VII as a Displacement of Conflict*, 6 TEMP. POL. & CIV. RTS. L. REV. 1–54 (1996).

22. For a description of how legal advisors have been indicted for aiding and abetting corporate noncompliance in relation to health care fraud and abuse, *see* N. Bilimoria, *Lawyers Beware of Criminal Health Care Fraud: What Attorneys Can Learn from the Kansas City Health Care Attorney Indictments*, 11:4 THE HEALTH LAW. 8–11 (1999). In this case the attorney was not ultimately convicted.

23. *See* A. Silverstein, *Ethical Issues Facing Corporate Counsel*, ANTITRUST 18–22 (Fall 1998).

24. HEALTH CARE COMPLIANCE ASSOCIATION, CODE OF ETHICS FOR HEALTH CARE COMPLIANCE PROFESSIONALS (1999).

25. DEPARTMENT OF HEALTH AND HUMAN SERVICES, OFFICE OF INSPECTOR GENERAL'S COMPLIANCE PROGRAM GUIDANCE FOR HOSPITALS, n.35 (Feb. 1998). HHS makes similar comments in its compliance program guidance for other health care providers, including Clinical Laboratories (Aug. 1998), Nursing Facilities (Mar. 2000), and Medicare + Choice Organizations Offering Coordinated Care Plans (Nov. 1999).

26. The U.S. Federal Sentencing Guidelines supports this principle by providing that specific individuals must be assigned with responsibility to oversee compliance within the organization and that they must be of a high level in order for a compliance program to qualify an organization for mitigating credits on sentencing. U.S. Sentencing Commission, *Sentencing of Organizations*, U.S. SENTENCING GUIDELINES MANUAL Ch. 8 (1993).

27. *See* G. Imperato, *Internal Investigations, Government Investigations, Whistleblower Concerns: Techniques to Protect Your Health Care Organization*, 51 ALA. L. REV. 210–11 (1999).

28. R.C. Park, *Ethical Challenges: The Dual Role of Attorney-Employee as Inside Corporate Counsel*, 22:3 HAMLINE L. REV. 783–96 (1999).

29. *See* J.E. Murphy, *Enhancing the Compliance Officer's Authority: Preparing an Employment Contract*, 11:6 ETHIKOS 5 (May/June 1998).

30. *See* R.C. Park, *Ethical Challenges: The Dual Role of Attorney-Employee as Inside Corporate Counsel*, 22:3 HAMLINE L. REV. 783–96 (1999).

31. *See* L. MAY, THE SOCIALLY RESPONSIVE SELF: SOCIAL THEORY AND PROFESSIONAL ETHICS 119–22 (1996).

CHAPTER 7

When Professional Standards Conflict: Conflicts between Law, Ethics, and Self-Interest in Cases of Self-Disclosure

Jan C. Heller

> The decision to follow the OIG's suggested [Provider Self-Disclosure] Protocol rests exclusively with the provider. . . . [T]he OIG can offer only limited guidance on what is inherently a case-specific judgment.[1]
>
> Department of Health and Human Services,
> Office of the Inspector General

INTRODUCTION

Professionals are largely distinguished by the trust placed in them to make appropriate professional judgments.[2] They earn this trust by being trained, examined, certified, and sometimes licensed in highly specialized fields or bodies of knowledge, and then by employing that knowledge in making judgments about specific cases in ways that advance the good of their clients, their employing organizations, their professions, and society generally.[3] Professionals are said to be acting with integrity when they consistently make appropriate professional judgments over time and space.

The routine cases about which professionals must make judgments are usually addressed without hesitation. As important as they may be, in routine cases neither the judgment nor the integrity of professionals is at issue. Think of experienced physicians or attorneys who, after years of supervised education and specialized practice, are seeing similar cases day after day. Although they always need to be alert for the surprising or particularly difficult case that might appear, these physicians and attorneys have learned to make judgments about highly complex matters—to interpret a set of symptoms or facts so as to prescribe a certain treatment or to recommend a certain legal course of action—often rather easily and with little uncertainty. Some cases, however, are what can be described as "conflicted" cases, and judgments about these cases are not so easily made. Conflicted cases can sometimes leave professionals doubting their competency to make appropriate judgments and wondering if they are being forced to compromise their integrity, no matter what they do.

Health care compliance professionals (HCCPs) also face conflicted cases. And, to the extent that they expect to be accorded the same trust that members of traditional professions have come to enjoy, they also must make consistently appropriate judgments about conflicted cases. This chapter uses cases of self-disclosure to illustrate how HCCPs can learn to recognize and respond to conflicted cases in ways that do not compromise their integrity. Cases of self-disclosure are taken to be paradigmatic examples of the conflicted cases faced by HCCPs, and exploring them will help HCCPs develop the conceptual tools needed to make their judgments competently and with their integrity intact.[4] (Cases of self-disclosure also have complex legal and financial dimensions that will be discussed only insofar as they help illustrate the conflicts they create.) The discussion begins by proposing a standard of competency for HCCPs facing conflicted cases.

A COMPETENCY STANDARD FOR CONFLICTED CASES: THE FOUR Rs

What should society, peers, employing organizations, and clients expect of HCCPs when they face a conflicted case; that is, for what level of competency should they be held accountable? It is suggested here that HCCPs address this question by adapting and adopting a standard of competency similar to the one developed for the Providence Health System (called "The Four Rs of Ethics").[5] It is easy to remember and it captures the essential skills required of HCCPs when facing a conflicted case. This standard requires HCCPs to *recognize* the conflicted case as such, that is, as a conflicted case, and to *respond* to it appropriately. Responding appropriately means that HCCPs will either *resolve* the conflict presented by the case or *refer* it to more experienced professionals or other relevant bodies for advice, guidance, and resolution.

This said, it should be immediately obvious that this standard of competency is a procedural standard. That is, it tells HCCPs what to do with a conflicted case, but it tells them nothing substantively about what distinguishes a conflicted case from a nonconflicted case, about what it means to resolve the conflict, or to whom they should refer it for help. Thus, this procedural standard must be augmented by additional education and experience. One source of guidance can be found in the Health Care Compliance Association's (HCCA) Code of Ethics for Health Care Compliance Professionals. The following sections introduce some of the conceptual distinctions that are required to interpret HCCA's Code of Ethics effectively.

LEARNING TO RECOGNIZE CONFLICTED CASES

A conflicted case may be defined generally as one in which the agent is obligated, at least in *prima facie* terms,[6] to choose between a number of contradictory or conflicting courses of action at the same time when, due to the circumstances of the case, only one course can in fact be chosen. Genuinely conflicted cases often cause HCCPs inner turmoil or perplexity because they cannot satisfy the conflicting obligations or requirements associated with the case, or can satisfy only some requirements at great cost to the others. There are at least four types of cases that HCCPs will consistently need to recognize and respond to appropriately. Two are not, strictly speaking, conflicted cases in the sense defined here, although in actual situations they easily can be mistaken for or transformed into conflicted cases, and two are genuinely conflicted.

The first type of case is one that presents HCCPs with a choice that is *clearly right or clearly wrong*. Outright fraud must be treated as a very serious case when it is discovered by compliance professionals, but it should not usually be viewed as a conflicted case in the sense defined here. Fraud is a form of stealing. Unless exceptional circumstances arise—such as the classic case in which a father steals food to keep his children from starving in the context of an unjust economic system—stealing is always wrong, both morally and legally. Moreover, when a person steals, he or she almost always knows that it is wrong, which is why fraud does not generally lead to inner turmoil or perplexity in the sense in which the terms are being used here. (It can lead to inner turmoil in the sense of leading to subjective guilt or in the sense of creating intense anxiety resulting from a fear of being discovered, but here inner turmoil refers to rational perplexity or confusion, for which professionals should not necessarily feel guilt.) Although HCCPs may be initially unsure in legal terms whether suspected fraud is actual fraud, cases of actual fraud are not genuinely conflicted because HCCPs know exactly how they ought to respond to them. The Code of Ethics for Health Care Compliance Professionals is clear about such cases. R1.4 states:

> When health care compliance professionals (HCCPs) become aware of any decision by their employing organization which, if implemented, would constitute misconduct, adversely affect the health of patients, residents or clients, or defraud the system, the professional shall: (a) refuse to consent to the decision; (b) escalate [the matter] to the highest governing authority, as appropriate; (c) if serious issues remain unresolved after exercising "a" and "b", consider resignation; and (d) report the decision to public officials when required by law.[7]

Now, although this HCCA standard addresses ongoing or future wrongdoing and does not directly address past misconduct,[8] the point here is that actual fraud simply cannot be promoted, condoned, or tolerated by HCCPs who want to gain or keep the public's trust, and this is widely acknowledged and accepted.

The second type of case is also not a conflicted case in the sense defined here, but it can be harder to recognize for what it is than cases that are clearly right or wrong. It can be harder to recognize because this second type of case can lead to self-deception on the part of professionals. It arises when choosing the right course of action *conflicts with the professional's self-interest*. Normally, of course, there is nothing morally or legally wrong with trying to advance one's self-interest, but it can become wrong when doing so conflicts with other moral or legal obligations.

Consider a case of *suspected* fraud, say, one in which there is reason to believe that the HCCP's employing organization has received improper overpayments for a number of years.[9]

> Case 1: You have been the compliance officer (CO) of your health system for two years, and have a reputation for being tough but fair in your treatment of employees and in your evaluation of potential compliance problems. The health system just acquired a small multihospital rural health system and somehow the "due diligence" efforts before the acquisition failed to uncover a problem with its cost reports. It now seems that an earlier

bond issue was used to pay off some debts that indirectly resulted in a net gain of $2.5 million. This gain was never reported, even though an audit had identified the problem, and it resulted in an increase in reimbursement from Medicare over the last 10 years. There is also evidence that the acquired entity's chief financial officer (CFO) knew of the problem through the audit and chose not to act on it.

Of course, whether the CFO of the acquired entity is actually guilty of fraud is certainly a question that should be investigated by competent counsel, and the acquiring entity would want to be sure that the problems with the cost reports were accurately assessed in financial terms by a reputable auditor or auditing firm. The recommendation to disclose the problem with the cost reports most likely would be made rather easily. Although it must be acknowledged that there is probably not a *general* legal obligation to self-disclose,[10] in this case it is likely that disclosure is in the interest of both the acquiring entity and the CO, as well as the right course of action ethically. As with the first type of case discussed earlier, HCCPs usually know without doubt that they are morally required to bring such cases to the attention of their superiors for referral to counsel.

Suppose, however, that this case were altered. Now, before the suspected fraud can be referred, suppose that the HCCP's superiors make it clear that they do not intend to refer the case to counsel, and that the professional's doing so will result in some personal or professional penalty (this threat need not be overtly stated, but could be subtly suggested in any number of ways). In such cases, choosing the right course of action can cost an HCCP a great deal, and under the pressure of these circumstances it is possible that he or she will inappropriately rationalize a decision to "go along" with his or her superiors. This professional may deceive him- or herself concerning the seriousness of the suspected fraud, or may try to convince him- or herself that he or she has done all that could be reasonably expected professionally by escalating the issue to the immediate superiors.

This type of case presents HCCPs with a genuine conflict (between taking the right course of action and their self-interest); however, again, it is not a case of conflicted obligations in the sense defined here. When professionals are confronted with cases that lead them to put what is clearly the right course of action against their own self-interest, professionals know (or, at least, ought to know) that they are both ethically and legally obligated to choose the right course of action. Although the stress such cases can create for professionals should not be minimized, it is just such stress that can lead to the self-deception against which professionals must guard.[11] The above-quoted rule from the HCCA's Code of Ethics is clear that, if necessary, the HCCP has a responsibility to escalate such matters to the highest governing body of the organization, and even to consider resignation and reporting the suspected fraud to public officials (if legally required). And, although this kind of a choice may not be professionally or psychologically easy, as it may have very negative consequences associated with it for HCCPs, it is exactly the kind of decision that is expected of them by the public. Professionals enjoy their status as professionals because they put the public's good above their employing organization's good and even above their own.[12] This, again, is in part what distinguishes them as professionals.

This said, it was mentioned earlier how such cases can be transformed into cases that are genuinely conflicted, and before going on this possibility should be considered. This transformed case is an example of the third type of case considered here. It is one of *conflicting ethical obligations or conflicting legal obligations*, that is, a case in which two or more ethical obligations conflict with each other, or two or more legal obligations conflict with each other. (The fourth type of case, one in which ethical obligations conflict with legal obligations, is considered below.)

There is at least anecdotal evidence that, in the years before the compliance movement gained momentum in the United States, health care executives often claimed (albeit, perhaps not publicly) that their decision to keep overpayments was *not*, in fact, a case of their self-interest going astray, but one of keeping funds that were justly "owed" them by an unjust reimbursement system. This claim was complicated by the public's and the government's expectation that the uninsured and underinsured patients would be treated by health care organizations regardless of the patients' ability to pay or regardless of the ability of the organization to be reimbursed for the treatment from other sources. Thus, it was claimed, the overpayments were sometimes not disclosed as a way of bringing some justice or equity to an unjust reimbursement system. If this claim could be empirically demonstrated, the above case of suspected fraud might be transformed from a case of self-interest into the third type of case, namely, one where the professional seems to be ethically or legally required to choose between two or more courses of action at the same time and in fact is able to choose only one.

In this transformed case, the HCCP, as part of the executive team, is not deceiving him- or herself about the decision to "go along" with the organization's other leaders, but is in a situation that is at least arguably analogous to the father who is stealing bread for his starving children in the context of an unjust economic system. The health care organization could claim, again arguably, that it is keeping the overpayments not to advance its interests, but to address the health care needs of the uninsured and underinsured through, say, cross-subsidization. The context of an unjust economic system is crucial in making this case into one of justified stealing, for the agent must be able to claim that no other ethically or legally acceptable course of action is available. The conflicted choice with which the health care executives are now confronted is between doing business honestly, and thereby *not* addressing the needs of the uninsured and the underinsured in their community, and doing business dishonestly, and thereby addressing the needs of the uninsured and the underinsured in their community. Indeed, these executives might view themselves as the contemporary health care equivalent of Robin Hood.

A decision-making process that can be used to resolve such conflicts will be developed below, but first a question should be asked: Is the recharacterization of the case of suspected fraud itself justified? This is an important question to ask in analyzing any case, for what amounts to a "presenting conflict" may, on reflection, not be an actual conflict or the most important one that the decision makers should be addressing.

In any event, this case has now been transformed into one that can be better characterized as a case of "gaming the system." Gaming the system is often practiced both for self-interested and for ethical reasons, and thus it is sometimes very hard for outside observers to decide the motives of the agents involved. For their motives to be judged as ethically acceptable, the health care executives—and the HCCP among them—would need to demonstrate empirically that the overpaid funds not returned to Medicare actually went to treat the uninsured and underinsured *and* that they had not themselves benefited as a result of the decision, say, by receiving a bonus or realizing an increase in occupational status for increasing the overall income of the organization. They may also need to bear the consequences of their choice, like those involved in civil disobedience.

Yet, some observers may care less about these executives' motives and more about other ways of evaluating this conduct. For instance, one could ask about the ability of their actions to be "generalized" in any example of gaming the system. In other words, would the consequences of gaming the system in this particular case be justified if *all* health care executives made similar choices in similar cases? (In fact, the generalizing of this practice may have led to the decision of the U.S. government to direct its compliance efforts toward the health care industry, as the costs of health care were spiraling out of control.) Gaming the system also can be judged by what is often called a "publicity test." Would these executives want this practice to be discussed, with their names associated with the discussion, on national television or in their community's papers? It is unlikely. Indeed, their public silence around this practice could be evidence that blatant self-interest is in fact being exercised or that these executives are truly deceiving themselves about their own motives. In any case, it is suggested here that gaming the system is generally wrong because, over time, it usually leads to worse consequences for everyone, but especially for the patients it is ostensibly supposed to help. In the end, gaming the system is hard to justify, ethically or legally, in part because it is so difficult to separate self-interest and genuine concern for others in such cases.

The fourth type of case is also genuinely conflicted in the sense defined earlier. In the fourth type of case, the professional faces *conflicting obligations of different types*, say, where ethical obligations conflict with legal obligations.[13] These cases can be difficult to resolve, as it is often is not clear whether commonly accepted ethical requirements should "trump" the specific requirements of the law, or vice versa. In any event, cases of self-disclosure will often present such conflicts to HCCPs. Indeed, a conflict of the fourth type could easily arise in cases of self-disclosure if a moral presumption is granted in favor of disclosing suspected wrongdoing when it appears that there is at least no general legal obligation to self-disclose and when the HCCA Code of Ethics requires disclosure when legally required. Moreover, this type of conflict can be further complicated by the interest-based incentives built into the U.S. Sentencing Guidelines,[14] as the long-term interests of the HCCP's employing organization to self-disclose can sometimes conflict with its short-term interests.

With this background, consider now the following case of self-disclosure:

Case 2: Two years ago your health care organization instituted a new compliance program and you were promoted one year ago from within the organization to become its first CO. As you are coming on board, you learn that the organization's first comprehensive risk-assessment revealed that your fiscal intermediary (FI) has been consistently overpaying your Medicare claims. You bring the matter to your CFO and, to your surprise, he tells you that he's been aware of the problem for some time; in fact, he tells you that his repeated attempts to correct the problem with the FI have not resolved the issue—the FI reports that its investigations did not uncover any systematic overpayment. The CFO concludes by saying, "You can report this to the government if you want to, but as far as I'm concerned, it's the FI's problem. If they can't fix their own mistakes, we should just keep the money and forget about it."

Compared with Case 1, this case presents a somewhat more complicated set of facts and issues for the HCCP. Here, the purported wrongdoing is ongoing and thus all the more urgent. Moreover, both the CO and CFO agree that this case should be disclosed, but they disagree as to whom the disclosure should be made, the FI or a government official. The CFO is clearly frustrated (perhaps justifiably) with the FI's inability or unwillingness to address the issue and to do so in a timely way. Nevertheless, this is a case in which the CO knows that the right course of action is to disclose the problem, both for ethical and for self-interested reasons (for the health care organization will bear final responsibility for the problem, not the FI, if it is discovered by a government investigator). Again, however, although there may be a legal obligation to return the money, there is probably no general legal obligation to disclose in this case; hence, the conflict. It is also a case in which the CO also might try to discover whether the CFO is somewhat misled by his self-interest. Indeed, as discussed earlier, this is exactly the kind of case that may have been ignored or discounted by hospital executives a few years ago, believing, like the CFO, either that they had done all that was ethically required or that it was permissible to follow what was sometimes purported to be the common practice among their colleagues, namely, to ignore such problems. But the overpayment presumably does not belong to this organization, and however much the CFO is motivated by enlightened self-interest or by a commendable loyalty to the organization or the community, the hard edge of the law can expose such rationalizations for what they are and remind professionals of their responsibilities. Here the law functions as a teacher as well as a guide to action.

RESPONDING TO THE CONFLICT

The last case considered here is a more interesting and complex case, and an example of the fourth type of conflicted case. This case will be discussed, however, in the context of a decision-making process in order to illustrate how the process might be useful in resolving such cases.

> Case 3: A recent "risk-assessment" of your laboratory practices results in a finding that your laboratory may have been inappropriately "bundling" certain tests between 1990 and 1994, at which time the laboratory manager learned of Operation Bad Bundle and discontinued the practice. As the CO, however, you are trying to decide whether and to whom to disclose the problem. Your estimates tell you that the overpayment was relatively small and there is no evidence that would lead you to think that the organization is currently the target of an investigation. Moreover, your legal counsel is telling you that there is no compelling legal duty to disclose this overpayment, and she recommends you do nothing, at least for now. But your chief executive officer (CEO) is new and he is highly motivated to keep the organization above suspicion "on his watch." He wants to disclose the overpayment and repay it, no matter how small. Everyone is afraid, however, that the disclosure will result in additional investigations, the results of which are unpredictable.

Now, assuming HCCPs can, in fact, recognize the genuine and multiple conflicts embedded in this rather complex case, the most important action they can take is to respond appropriately to them. Responding appropriately means, first, that professionals should not ignore such cases. Admittedly, ignoring significantly conflicted cases is not likely to happen due to a discrete decision, but is much more likely to happen as a result of the press of other, competing responsibilities. Nevertheless, ignoring them might not only be unethical and a breach of the CO's responsibilities, it might also be very short-sighted and contrary to a professional's self-interest. Second, responding appropriately means that professionals will either resolve the conflict(s) in the case or refer it to others who can resolve it. To resolve the conflict(s) means that a course of action is chosen that satisfies the conflicting obligations embedded in the case or, if this is not possible, that a choice is made that represents the "right" or "best" course of action, all things considered. In actual cases, it is likely that HCCPs will involve a number of other decision makers who, together, will decide either to resolve or refer the case. And, of course, resolving a case of self-disclosure means deciding whether to refer it to government officials.

One way to resolve such cases quickly is simply to allow one perspective or set of rules to "trump" the other perspectives or sets of rules. For example, the organization's code of conduct may claim that the organization's employees and associates are committed to the "highest ethical standards," and the CO or the CEO may realize that any breach of those standards, should it become public, will undermine the compliance program's credibility with employees and the public. The CO might argue that such factors should lead decision makers to override the legal counsel's opinion. Admittedly, in some cases this may be justified. But in more complex cases, it can be helpful to stop and take some time to think about the possible or probable consequences of a variety of alternative responses. The decision makers may end up at the same place, but they should have more confidence in their decision. It is recommended that such a discipline be utilized with this case.

In trying to resolve complex or novel conflicted cases, it is often useful to follow a more or less formal decision-making process. A decision-making process is simply a set of steps to be followed or points to be considered before deciding what course of action to take with a conflicted case; essentially, it is a way of making sure that "all the bases are covered." It is important to realize, however, that no decision process can *guarantee* the right or best decision; it is not an algorithm, but merely an aid to human judgment, which remains fallible.

This said, at least the following six steps can be used in a decision-making process involving conflicts like those discussed here. Step 1 is actually used as a step prior to beginning the process, in order to decide whether to resolve the case or refer it to others for resolution (a decision to refer can be made at any point in the process, if the decision makers decide that they cannot resolve the conflicts or if they are not the decision makers who ought to be making the choice).

If the HCCP chooses to resolve the conflict in the case, Steps 2 through 4 involve analyzing the conflict(s) inherent in the case. Step 2 requires the HCCP to identify all relevant decision makers and to facilitate their input. This can be done face to face, on a telephone or video conference, or in some combination of these, and it can sometimes require very little time, although at other times it can require multiple meetings. The effort should be made to identify *all* relevant decision makers both because complex cases usually require experts from various fields and because too few or the wrong decision makers can bias the outcome in ways that could be detrimental for those affected by the decision. This group can also grow or shrink as the case dictates. A presupposition of participation as a decision maker is the intention to choose the right course of action, to the extent the right course of action can be discovered or created. If it is learned that certain decision makers are not interested in choosing the right course of action, the group may need to exclude them; indeed, it may be that they are part of the problem under consideration. For Case 3, the relevant decision makers are, at a minimum, the HCCP (the CO in this case), the legal counsel, and the CEO. Other likely participants are the CFO and perhaps a board representative. The laboratory manager, and anyone else who might be needed for background information or for predicting whether other investigations are likely should they choose to self-disclose, should probably not be included as decision makers, but rather as persons who supply relevant information to the decision makers.

Step 3 requires the decision makers to define and agree on a definition of the conflict(s) in a given case. This is important for a number of reasons. First, as was mentioned earlier, not all conflicts that present themselves ("presenting conflicts") are the most important conflicts in a case. In other words, the conflicts that bring the decision makers together might not, on reflection, be the key conflicts on which they ought to focus. Complex cases often have "layers" that need to be "peeled back" and analyzed carefully. The HCCP who calls the group together needs to recognize only that there is some conflict in the case that should be analyzed, but the relevant decision makers must decide together whether the presenting conflict is the actual conflict or the most important one for their consideration. Second, the decision makers should agree on a definition of the conflicts so that they do not work at cross-purposes to each other; this is merely good group dynamics and important for the efficiency of the work. Unfortunately, however, agreeing on the conflicts in question is not always easy, and sometimes takes a great deal of prior information gathering and discussion; at other times it will be obvious to everyone.

Case 3 probably has all four types of conflict in it that have been considered in this chapter. First, if the inappropriate bundling was actually done, which seems likely, it has been acknowledged internally as clearly wrong and has been discontinued. The second issue of the organization's self-interest is not as clear, however. It is simply not obvious whether it is in the interest of the organization to disclose the inappropriate bundling. On the one hand, the overpayment is very small and there is no evidence that the organization is a target of an investigation. On the other hand, additional investigations could be very detrimental to the interests of the organization. Third, the possible negative consequences to the organization from disclosure could lead to a genuine ethical conflict for the CO: the CO's laudable ethical inclinations to disclose the overpayment could conflict with the CO's obligations of loyalty to the organization. If unexpected findings detrimental to the organization arise during a subsequent investigation, it could be argued that the CO should have anticipated such findings and disclosed these results as well, at least saving the penalties associated with nondisclosure. And fourth, the CO's and the CEO's ethical inclinations to self-disclose conflict with the legal counsel's recommendations that nothing be done in this case.

Which of these conflicts should be regarded as the most important? This could be debated, of course, but it appears that the CO's and the CEO's conflict with the legal counsel's recommendation is the key conflict in this case (and an example of the fourth type of conflict discussed here); resolving the other conflicts contributes to resolving this conflict.

Step 4 requires decision makers to list the alternative choices available to address the conflict(s) identified in Step 3. This can be a difficult step from an empirical perspective, for not only does it require that the decision makers list all the affected stakeholders [15] under each alternative, it also requires them to try to predict each alternative's effects on the stakeholders. In Case 3, there are essentially two alternative choices, to self-disclose or not, and the stakeholders are the same under each alternative. The organizational leaders (the CO, CEO, and legal counsel, and perhaps other officers and board members of the organization) and some employees (the laboratory manager and perhaps the laboratory staff) would obviously be affected by the choice; the organization itself, with its other employees and associates, as well as the patients and larger community served by the organization, could be affected if the choice results in penalties significant enough to threaten the economic survival of the organization; and, finally, those citizens whose Medicare taxes paid for the overpayments, and Medicare itself, an important institution in this country, could be affected.

When predicting effects on stakeholders, decision makers should not rush too quickly to evaluate those effects. This is especially true for complex cases and why this process should be viewed to this point primarily as an analytical exercise, not an evaluative one. It other words, the probable or actual effects (to the extent these are possible to predict) on the stakeholders should be described without deciding at this step whether these effects are good or bad, or whether they should be regarded as benefits or harms, relative to the affected stakeholders. The evaluation of the identified effects is done at Step 5. Also, predicting effects on certain stakeholders, like organizations or institutions, can require extensive information gathering. It will be shown that this proves to be true in Case 3. Finally, if constraints of confidentiality permit, it is important to interview stakeholders who are affected, for the middle level managers or line employees who are not included in the decision making group may have information or perspectives that upper level decision makers incorrectly assume they know or can represent accurately.

This said, decision makers should imagine the affected stakeholders as grouped in concentric circles, with those most affected being on the inner circles and those least affected being on the outer circles. It is sometimes helpful to begin predicting effects by considering the least affected early; they can sometimes (but not always, so be careful) be "discounted" in particular cases. In Case 3, decision makers might legitimately discount the effects of the laboratory bundling on U.S. citizens as taxpayers and on Medicare as an institution, if their laboratory manager's initial investigation proves to be accurate. One way to test this (before an actual self-disclosure to government officials, who may decide otherwise, of course) is to consider whether the government's costs related to processing the self-disclosure would actually be greater than the overpayment itself. If the overpayment is small enough, it may not be worth the government's effort. But part of this calculation in Case 3 involves coming to terms with the confusing implications of the conflicts around self-interest. This case of inappropriate bundling may not be worth pursuing, but if the government decided that this case indicated a general practice by the organization, it might initiate an investigation in order to uncover other problems.

Predicting the effects on the other stakeholders probably turns on this same calculation, that is, on the likelihood of further government investigations if disclosure is made (and, it must be remembered, investigations can always be initiated without disclosure), and the likelihood, if the government investigation were initiated, that something unethical or illegal would actually be discovered. Assuming no other problems would be uncovered by an investigation, self-disclosure would have little effect on any of the stakeholders in this case. (A possible exception to this generalization might be the employee(s) who misinterpreted the laboratory coding procedures in the first place. If that person(s) is still employed by the organization, that stakeholder might face some degradation in rank or loss in status.) There is no evidence of intentional fraud in this case. As soon as the inappropriate bundling was discovered, it was discontinued. Thus, it is unlikely that criminal charges would be brought against the organizational leaders or the board. The civil penalties leveled for such a small overpayment would need to be considered, but presumably they are small enough that the legal counsel has determined that the risk of nondisclosure is worth taking. In the end, then, the magnitude of the effects of this choice to self-disclose or not turn on the unknown probability that the government will investigate and that it will find other issues when it does so.

If this analysis is correct, then it can be concluded that the only way to remove or reduce this unknown probability is to initiate an *internal* investigation. This could be costly in terms of time and money, but it is probably less costly than waiting for the government to do it and having undisclosed problems discovered in the process. (The investigation should also be completed in a timely way, of course, as the government could later view delay negatively.) Thus, one recommendation the decision makers could make at this point is to stop the decision-making process at Step 4 and delay the decision on whether to self-disclose until they have more information. This is the only way to address the confusion around the question of the organization's self-interest. This is a legitimate question, and should not be discounted when considering the ethical and legal issues involved in a case. If an internal investigation reveals no additional problems, then Step 5, evaluating the alternatives (which should be done on the basis of the organization's values, the professional's personal and professional values, and ethical and legal or regulatory standards) may be accomplished very easily. With little risk to the organization, the ethical inclinations of the CO and CEO could be followed and the inappropriate bundling disclosed, regardless of the fact that there may be no compelling legal obligation to do so. In this scenario, the CO's and the CEO's ethical inclinations essentially trump the legal counsel's advice, for although there is no legal obligation to disclose the problem, the decision makers now know there is no good reason not to disclose. It could even help them build credibility with the government should this be needed later.

On the other hand, if an internal investigation does in fact reveal further significant problems, the interest-based incentives built into the Sentencing Guidelines might also lead the decision makers to decide for self-disclosure in any case, and with the support of the legal counsel. With knowledge of further problems, it is likely that the penalties associated with discovery by the government would be great enough to warrant self-disclosure, and this too would overcome the conflict between the ethical and legal obligations. Step 6 instructs the decision makers merely to implement whatever decision they make, to communicate it as necessary, and to follow up on it, especially if they need to address any remaining negative consequences for stakeholders.

Case 3 is interesting, then, for what it reveals about choosing among alternatives. When the analysis is done thoroughly—in this case, requiring the decision makers to go back and do a laborious internal investigation—it is often true that the resolution presents itself. It is also often true that the ethical and legal conflicts that loom large in the given case are resolved, not by hard ethical or legal analysis (although this is sometimes required), but by additional empirical information. What makes such cases truly hard is when that additional information is not available, is not reliable, or is ambiguous. In such situations, the conflict between ethics and law may not be resolvable, and decision makers will be forced to decide whether their moral obligations are more important than their legal obligations (happily, they will usually not conflict, but they can). Most likely, this choice will turn less on the rational and empirical factors in a given case, and more on the characters of the decisions makers and of the organization. Nevertheless, such irremediable conflicts are truly "hard choices," and may not admit to "resolution" in the sense discussed here.

CONCLUSION

This chapter employed cases of self-disclosure to illustrate four different types of conflicted cases about which HCCPs must make appropriate judgments. It was shown that two of these conflicted cases—those that involve choices about courses of action that are clearly right or wrong, and those that involve some choice that promotes or harms the self-interests of the professional—are not genuinely conflicted in the sense defined here, that is, in the sense that they lead to conflicting obligations and to genuine rational perplexity or inner turmoil. The other two—those that involve conflicting ethical obligations or conflicting legal obligations, and those that involve conflicts between ethics and law—can be a source of much perplexity and inner turmoil for conscientious professionals. As a minimum standard of competency, it is suggested that professionals should recognize and respond appropriately to such cases, and that responding appropriately means either resolving the conflict(s) in the case or referring it. To help professionals resolve them, a six-step decision-making process was outlined as an aid to making professional judgments in conflicted cases. Following this decision-making process will not guarantee that the right or best decision is made, but it should increase the likelihood that this will happen.

NOTES

1. Department of Health and Human Services, Office of the Inspector General, Publication of the OIG's Provider Self-Disclosure Protocol, 63 Fed. Reg. 58,400 (1998).
2. "Judgment" here means the process of bringing information, experience, and the relevant criteria to bear on a situation or case so as to form a considered opinion. This process also may be described as an act of "discernment."
3. *See* Chapter 1, *Professional Ethical Development in Health Care Compliance*.
4. For a more extensive discussion of the conflicts introduced here, see J.C. Heller, *Framing Healthcare Compliance in Ethical Terms: A Taxonomy of Moral Choices*, 11:4 HEC FORUM 345–57 (1999). Some of the distinctions discussed in this chapter were first presented in this article, and permission by the editor, Dr. Stuart Spicker, to use some of that material here is gratefully acknowledged.
5. PROVIDENCE HEALTH SYSTEM, RECOGNIZING AND RESOLVING VALUE CONFLICTS: AN ETHICAL DECISION MAKING PROCESS FOR PHS LEADERS (2000).
6. The qualification *prima facie* is used as a way of signaling that what might be called the "presenting conflict" in a given case may, on reflection, not be an actual conflict or may not be the most important one in the case. As discussed below, part of the analysis of the conflict involves determining exactly where to focus one's concern.
7. HEALTH CARE COMPLIANCE ASSOCIATION, CODE OF ETHICS FOR HEALTH CARE COMPLIANCE PROFESSIONALS (1999).
8. This distinction between past, present, and future wrongdoing can be relevant in the cases of self-disclosure discussed below. Whether the wrongdoing is past, present, or future is a fact that is often irrelevant in an ethical analysis of a case (the determination that an action is wrong ethically does not usually turn on *when* it happened or happens), but can be relevant in a legal analysis. An action that is determined to be legally wrong may or may not turn on the time the action happens; nevertheless, attorneys are obligated not to disclose the *past* wrongdoing of their clients, but may, under certain circumstances, be obligated to disclose *present* or planned, *future* wrongdoing. This interesting qualification is owed to Joseph E. Murphy.

9. Case 1, and the cases below labeled Case 2 and Case 3, are adapted from G.M. Luce and H. O'Shea, Self-Disclosure for Healthcare Organizations Program Materials, presented at a Voluntary Hospitals of America (VHA) Compliance Officers Affinity Group Meeting (June 24, 1999). The text is changed from the original. Permission to use these cases is gratefully acknowledged.

10. The Bureau of National Affairs, Inc., *Voluntary Disclosure*, 2600.09 BNA HEALTH LAW & BUSINESS SERIES 2600:0901–:0916 (Dec. 1999). It should be noted, however, that this same source claims "there may be specific statutes or regulations that compel a health care provider to report violations of the law of which the provider becomes aware." *See id.* at 2600.0902.

11. For an in-depth discussion of stress and its effects, *see* Chapter 10, *Stress Management for Compliance Professionals.*

12. In making this statement, it is assumed that the compliance professional is *not* the organization's legal counsel. If the same person occupies these two roles, the case could be complicated by the attorney–client protections.

13. Ethical and legal obligations are not, of course, the only type of obligations that exist or that can conflict. One also could consider political, fiscal, and religious obligations that, given certain circumstances, could easily conflict with either ethical or legal obligations, or both.

14. U.S. SENTENCING GUIDELINES MANUAL (1987).

15. Stakeholders can be persons, organizations, or institutions affected by the choice in question. The terms "organization" and "institution" are often used interchangeably, but there are differentiated here. A given health care facility is or is not part of an organization, whereas the health care delivery system in the United States is an institution.

CHAPTER 8

Protecting Yourself and Your Profession

Joseph E. Murphy

WHY COMPLIANCE PROFESSIONALS NEED PROTECTION

Those who perform in-house compliance work face a daunting task. They know the work is difficult, and that there is likely to be ongoing controversy about the things that they propose. They may feel uneasy about their tasks, but in the press of daily business may not have much time to think about the risk side of their positions. However, as is discussed here, the in-house compliance position is one that is unusually risky; serious consideration needs to be given to recognizing and minimizing the risks.

Several elements, in particular, contribute to the difficulty and risk of the in-house compliance position. First, there is the difficult feat of pursuing the three roles addressed in Chapter 3: consulting, policing, and managing.[1] The compliance professional needs to keep close to the client to master the consulting role. This familiarity with the client's business also makes the professional more effective in the managing and policing roles. Thus, the professional will want to attend important management meetings where key decisions are made affecting the business and related compliance risks. Yet the compliance professional must also maintain a strong degree of objectivity and independence to do an effective job in the policing and issue-spotting roles. Like those in the legal profession, compliance professionals need to be able to step away from the client's day-to-day business perspective and see business conduct in a different light. The compliance professional must be able to see a business proposal with the eyes of an outside skeptic. How would the government, the press, or an injured consumer view a proposed course of conduct with the benefit of hindsight? The compliance professional also needs to be free to examine allegations of past misconduct without being led astray by pleas to protect those who were involved in wrongdoing.

As pointed out in Chapter 3, this creates conflict. The compliance professional may be the only one holding out for strong discipline, or refusing to close an investigation until fundamental changes are made in how business is conducted. This conflict can breed ill will toward the compliance professional. Other managers who may expect the compliance professional to be a "team player" may view the compliance professional as possibly playing for the opposing team.

In addition to the conflicts inherent in the multifaceted role of compliance professional, there is also conflict and risk built into any internal policing role that seeks to ensure compliance with externally imposed standards of conduct. This conflict is rooted in the very nature of organizations. As such, each organization exists to serve a purpose. That is why people join together in organizations. In the case of a business, the purpose starts with making money. This may not be the only purpose, however, and this is not to take the cynical and myopic view that profit is the only reason for a business to exist. But whatever the purpose or purposes may be, they are the drivers for the organization's conduct.

The compliance professional has the function and duty of preventing and detecting wrongdoing. When the wrongdoing targets the company, such as employee theft from the company, or it disrupts efficient operation of the business, such as sexual harassment, then the company's and the professional's interests may be perfectly aligned. But preventing wrongdoing may well create conflict with organizational objectives, at least in the short run. It may be, for example, that earnings are down at a critical point in the organization's business. There may be a push to defer costs, such as those associated with environmental management, or to increase revenues through questionable accounting techniques. The compliance professional must resist unethical or illegal steps that would ease the short-term pain for managers of the organization.

Nor does the conflict end at that level. In any complex organization there will be potential conflicts among the sub-units of the organization. A successful compliance program needs to reach all employees in all units of the organization. Tagging one unit with additional compliance expenses, such as expensive safety apparatus, can add to tensions with that business unit. Thus, even though the parent company may recognize that compliance is good for the overall organization and its shareholders, the results may not be as positive for any particular business unit that perceives that it is bearing a disproportionate impact.

These internal political factors, difficult as they may be, have less intense downside implications for the compliance professional when compared with the next factor, the legal risks of compliance work.[2] The position of compliance professional is, in a sense, intended to be in harm's way. The compliance function exists, in part, to detect and respond to wrongdoing. If there is illegal conduct such as the bribery of officials, price fixing, or the distribution of dangerously defective products, then this is where the compliance professional is supposed to be. One need only consider the job functions associated with compliance work.[3] Compliance includes conducting audits to detect misconduct. If there is an indication of wrongdoing, then the compliance professional is there to participate in investigations of the alleged improper activity. If misconduct is discovered, then the compliance professional takes on a role in disciplining those involved. When the matter is serious enough, the compliance professional arranges to inform government prosecutors about the misconduct.

These difficult tasks are combined with the fact that compliance deals with risky and often complex legal areas. The list of danger areas is extensive,[4] including discrimination and harassment, environmental crimes, False Claims Act violations, patient mistreatment, and patient and employee privacy issues.

When problems are uncovered in these areas, the compliance program and its personnel exist, in part, to be available as evidence in contested legal proceedings. One of the motivating factors for companies to have compliance programs is to be able to obtain more lenient treatment from the government and the legal system. Whether trying to convince a U.S. Attorney not to indict, or a jury not to impose punitive damages,[5] if the bona fides of a program are in issue, it falls to the compliance professionals to prove the company's case.

Of course, the existence and effectiveness of the compliance program come into issue at the riskiest possible time, namely, after a violation has been discovered and the government and/or other adversaries are already suspicious. Everything about the program is likely to be examined carefully for defects. There may still be a tendency to assume that if wrongdoing occurred in a company, then managers were either "asleep at the switch" or were part of the wrongdoing.

In this environment, what risks confront the compliance professional? In the United States, where employment at will is still the rule, a compliance professional, like most other employees, faces the prospect of being terminated whenever his or her boss is displeased. Entire compliance units could be downsized, outsourced, or eliminated completely as part of cost cutting or a change in corporate strategy.

The compliance professional has special vulnerability in this environment. Like many staff groups, the compliance organization is a cost element, not a revenue generator. When implemented the right way, an effective compliance program can reduce costs and even be part of the marketing effort to customers, but it is still relatively rare for management to be that enlightened in the approach to compliance. What exacerbates the risk is the fact that the compliance manager is playing the policing role, and has a significant risk of getting on the wrong side of important people in the business.

Compliance professionals do not need to be terminated to be rendered ineffective or punished for doing their jobs too aggressively. A more subtle approach uses downgrades, marginalization, and disempowerment. One technique is to "enhance" or expand the scope of responsibilities of the compliance professional to include other work that distracts attention and resources from compliance. This can include functions that are unwanted by other corporate departments, such as the maintenance of corporate policies on such mundane issues as attendance. It is also possible to exclude the compliance staff from key activities, such as forgetting to invite a compliance representative to meetings on proposed acquisitions or strategic planning.

Although the organizational political risks are serious, the greatest harm can come from contact with illegal conduct and the risk of actual or perceived involvement in such conduct. If a compliance professional is doing his or her job, then the person is likely to become aware of any illegal activity in the organization through such sources as audits, investigations, and helpline calls. Although proximity to misconduct is not an offense, the chances of being tainted by it are naturally greater for those who come into contact with it.[6]

In today's environment of heightened scrutiny of business conduct and the government's increased expectations of cooperation by companies, the mere failure to act or to report misconduct can be interpreted as improper involvement in it. For example, the government views with suspicion any company that discovers an internal violation of the False Claims Act and fails to report and refund any overcharge. Enforcement officials claim that such passivity is, itself, a violation of the act. As any criminal defense attorney knows, American prosecutors have enormous power in determining whether to bring charges against, or even whether to investigate, someone. The powers at their disposal—grand juries, search warrants, wire taps, press conferences, suspension of so-called privileges (for example, the ability to do business with the government)—mean that the process of punishment actually starts at the moment the prosecutor decides to pursue an individual. For a compliance professional, whose ability to be employed depends on being on the side of doing the right thing, the impact of an investigation can be career ending. The costs and time requirements in just the investigation stage also can be sufficient to disrupt the compliance professional's life. And this assumes that the professional is ultimately successful in avoiding conviction for an offense.

Compliance staff also face risk from private claims and civil litigation. For example, any employee engaged in conducting internal investigations and imposing discipline faces the risk of claims by a target of an investigation. Although the company, as a deep pocket, is the most likely target, individual employees are also subject to suit in tort actions. An employee who feels victimized by a compliance investigation may sue for defamation, based on any information that reached other employees or the outside world.[7] Thus, in the E. F. Hutton case,[8] the company had hired noted attorney Griffin Bell to conduct an investigation of employee misconduct. When the results of the investigation were gathered, the company issued a press announcement accusing specific managers of misconduct. As a result, the managers sued Griffin Bell for defamation.

A targeted employee may also make out a claim of interference with contract or economic advantage because the compliance activities caused loss of employment. If an investigation used aggressive techniques, courts also appear willing to entertain claims of invasion of privacy. In one case involving Kmart, the use of private investigators hired to mingle with employees and overhear any indications of misconduct was determined to be the basis for a claim of "intrusion on seclusion."[9]

Whether a litigating employee targets only the company, or includes the compliance professionals, all those involved are confronted with the costs of litigation, in terms of time and counsel fees. Even a successfully defended case, where the claims are ultimately thrown out before trial, involves costs that cannot be recouped from the other side. Actual out-of-pocket attorneys' fees, and the less tangible but nevertheless painful costs in terms of time, weigh on the defendants in such litigation.

If the compliance professional is not successful in defending such claims, there is the risk of damages payable to the employee who brings the claim. These can be substantial in terms of recovery of lost salary and other economic injury. In the context of tort actions, there is also the specter of punitive damages claims.

PROTECTION AND EMPOWERMENT

The risks for compliance professionals are as real as the regular parade of corporate misconduct stories in the daily newspapers. What direction does this suggest for the compliance professional? In this high-risk environment, compliance professionals have to be active participants, not passive observers. They cannot afford to work quietly, accepting whatever fate holds in store for them.

A first step is to be sure that they have the authority to conduct their jobs effectively. The relevant corporate authorizations and related documentation should reflect that they have the necessary authority to be effective in their corporations. Not only is this vital for the compliance professional, but it also serves a valuable purpose for the corporate client. All the steps described in this chapter to strengthen the compliance professional are also useful in the litigation context when the corporation is trying to demonstrate the effectiveness of its compliance program.

A logical starting point for this process is a resolution of the board of directors, or the highest governing authority in the organization. Starting here reflects the special role of the board. Unlike management, the board is not directly involved in day-to-day business matters, and can bring a fresh perspective to compliance matters. At least outside members of the board have other interests beyond the specific, short-term objectives of management. An outside director may be active in other companies, and not be as willing to accept short-term expedient actions that create legal risks. The director also faces higher-profile liability exposure. For the publicly traded company, the directors may well face shareowner derivative claims if they fail to implement and maintain an effective compliance program. In 1996, the Delaware Chancery Court warned directors that they faced this risk if they did not take into account the importance of having a system to keep them informed regarding corporate compliance.[10]

The board of directors' resolution should recite the company's commitment to compliance and ethical conduct. Beyond this, there is great value in having sufficient specificity to remove ambiguity about the strength of the compliance program. If the board specifies that it wants a program that is at least as good as the Sentencing Guidelines standards, that it is committed to best practices, and that it wants the company to be open about its program, this helps thwart objections that otherwise might arise from management. An example of a detailed resolution is set forth in Appendix 8–A of this chapter.

Among the issues that deserve detailed attention in the board's resolution is the question of reports on the program's progress and problems. Here it is advisable to require regular detailed reporting to the board. In some companies there is a reluctance to "weigh down the board" with detail. This mentality can result in perfunctory reports blandly assuring the board that "we are doing well and there are no unresolved problems." Boilerplating can easily replace the current, realistic insight that the board should have. Thus, the board could specify that it requires detailed reports on such specific areas as helpline calls, including trends; information on disciplinary cases; and tracking reports on open investigations. It is true that the board should not micromanage the business, but the detailed reporting helps drive the program forward. When this type of reporting system is in place, typically the time period immediately before the report is due will see an acceleration of compliance activity. At the same time, the reports should not "indict" the company or make unnecessary legal judgments that could be harmful in litigation. Reports to the board should have legal input, but should not be censored.

The board can also play a crucial role by holding the exclusive authority to elect or remove the compliance officer. Such a requirement is one clear sign that the compliance officer is actually a "high-level" company official, and not someone with an exalted title but no real substance. Another step that can empower the compliance professional is to require reporting to the board regarding any personnel changes made involving the compliance staff, not just the compliance officer. Such reporting can be required before any such changes can become effective, and the board can also mandate a written explanation for the changes. In the field of compliance, as may be true in other organizational matters, one of the most effective allies for the professional is inertia. If there is a requirement to go before the board in order to undermine the authority of the compliance staff, the potential for that to happen is greatly reduced.

In organizations, access to those who make the decisions is a form of power. The more filters there are to reach those decision makers, the more one's power is reduced.[11] Thus, another key element for empowerment of the compliance professional is direct access to the chief executive officer and to the board or audit committee. There may actually be a preference for access to the audit committee, and not just the board. At least for companies listed on the New York Stock Exchange, the audit committee must comprise nonmanagement directors. Access to this committee gives the compliance professional the ability to raise issues that might implicate senior management, without those senior managers being present in the first instance. This approach draws from the model of the internal auditors, who have access to the audit committee in executive session, with no managers present. Of course, if a company has a board-level compliance committee also comprising outside directors, this could serve the same role as the audit committee serves for the internal auditors.

There is also a value in making at least some elements of the reporting relationship mandatory. For example, a board or board committee could require the compliance officer to report any instance where an allegation is made involving any senior officer. It could also require a report in any case where the compliance officer requests access to employees or documents and is refused, or where there is a compliance recommendation that is not followed by management. This mandatory reporting requirement can substantially reduce the risk that managers will pose impediments to the compliance office. With a requirement that any such instances be reported to the board, management will resist only when it is prepared to give a convincing explanation to the board.

Although the reporting relationship can serve as a deterrent to harassment of the compliance officer and the compliance staff, it may not prove practical for the compliance officer to try to convene special meetings of the board or a board committee whenever issues arise. The logistics of this may present a practical impediment to the use of this resource. To make the reporting relationship more feasible, one practical approach is to have the board or committee delegate contact responsibility between scheduled meetings to one specific board member, such as the chair of the audit committee. In such cases the board member and the compliance officer should be comfortable with each other, with the compliance officer feeling free to call that contact to discuss developments on an ongoing, informal basis.

An additional documentary step that can help enhance the compliance professional's position, and at the same time provide another exhibit for the company to use in proving the substance of its program, is the position descriptions of the compliance staff. A position description can include reference to the board resolution that endorsed the program, and the professional's duty to execute that resolution. The description should be strong, and reflect the professional's plenary authority to carry out the compliance duties.

Board members and senior executives in large companies typically are protected by indemnification should they become the targets of litigation. The costs of defending such actions can be enormous. It is important for the compliance professional to know that the costs of litigation would be paid, or at least advanced by the company. Consideration should be given to providing such support, at least for the compliance officer, if not for the rest of the compliance staff. Companies may want to revise their bylaws, if necessary, to make such coverage applicable in the compliance context.

Perhaps an alternative to indemnification would be for the company to have insurance protecting the compliance personnel. There are limits on this alternative. In the case of criminal prosecution, such insurance might not be enforceable. Of course, if the compliance professional has in fact engaged in illegal conduct, the indemnification also would not apply.

All the protections previously discussed ultimately rely on the good faith of those associated with the company. Although it is true that those on the board may have a greater receptivity to compliance concerns than managers because of their liability exposure, this may not provide much protection in a board dominated by management. And in a closely held company there is not the counterbalance created by the threat of shareowner suits, stock exchange rules, and Securities and Exchange Commission (SEC) enforcement actions. This suggests consideration of a more legally rigorous form of protection, the employment contract.[12]

In the American corporate world, employment contracts are usually reserved for the true stars of the company, such as key managers in acquired companies. They are not typically offered to line and staff managers in the normal day-to-day business conditions. The existence of such a well-drafted contract could go far to establish clearly the compliance officer's authority. By giving the compliance officer the authority and degree of autonomy appropriate for the job, it can provide strong independence, and can be one of the few sources of protection in a privately owned company. It should be remembered, however, that, like all parts of a compliance program, there needs to be a fit with the culture of the company. Although durable protection is appropriate no matter what the current culture and leadership of the company, it can take great political skill to obtain a strong contract without offending other managers who do not have such protection.

What types of things should be included in the contract? Appendix 8–B contains a checklist that covers a variety of points. It may not be necessary to include each of these, but they can all be on the list of items to consider, depending on the circumstances of the company and what other protections are available.

In drafting such a contract, the compliance officer should obtain advice and assistance from competent legal counsel. But no matter how strong the language of the contract, it is important to remember that it is only a contract, and parties do break contracts. If management is unhappy with the compliance officer, it can elect to breach the contract and then pay damages in litigation. This is not a step likely to be taken lightly by management, however, because such litigation would open to public exposure, at a minimum, a highly embarrassing internal dispute in the sensitive area of compliance and ethics.

One potential alternative to the contract is for the compliance officer to negotiate a rich buy-out option. In this way the company could terminate the compliance officer, but would have to pay a large amount of money. For the company, this reduces the risk of embarrassing litigation. Although this may enhance the comfort level of the potential recipient of the money, it is obviously less effective in protecting society from organizational misconduct. In the contract arrangement, the deterrent to misconduct is the recognition that it may take ugly, newsworthy litigation to get rid of the compliance officer who objects to the misconduct. In the case of the buy-out, ejecting the compliance officer becomes strictly a matter of money, just like any other business decision. The buy-out arrangement may also raise skepticism among the compliance officer's staff, who are not likely to have a similar golden parachute, and may not have the sense that the compliance officer has quite the same incentive to remain in the trenches to fight the good fight.

To execute their responsibilities in an organization, compliance professionals need the necessary resources, and they especially need access to information about the organization's activities. Probably foremost on the list of needed resources is access to the legal staff on a priority basis. As noted earlier, the compliance staff has to work in some of the most complex and dangerous legal areas. They need to have access to legal expertise in those areas, from an attorney who understands the nature of compliance work.

In some companies this objective is achieved by the creation of a compliance counsel, an attorney who is the primary legal resource for the compliance program. Although the compliance officer should always have direct access to the company's general counsel, a staff attorney who knows the details of the compliance program can be an enormously important source of assistance and protection for the compliance staff. Also to be considered, although much more controversial, would be direct access to outside counsel, and even having separate counsel for the compliance officer. This is likely to happen only in cases where companies have already been prosecuted and the compliance office is really an independent monitor installed as part of a settlement agreement.

Access to legal counsel is a key starting point, but there are other groups whose assistance is important for the compliance office. Departments like human resources, security, auditing, and information technology all have resources and powers that are valuable for the functioning of the compliance office. Their availability and active participation in the compliance program can serve as vital support for the compliance effort.

In addition to access to key personnel, the compliance office, in its policing role, needs unobstructed access to all records, facilities, employees, managers, and officers throughout the company. Effective auditing and investigations are essential elements for a credible compliance program. Some government agencies, for example, expect to see unannounced audits to detect misconduct if the program is to have credibility with law enforcement.[13] These functions cannot be performed satisfactorily if parts of the business can insulate themselves from review. The model for this level of authority is the internal audit organization, which similarly would insist on the ability to review any part of the company's records and operations.

The reality of power in the organization has to be a starting point for the compliance professional, but there must also be an awareness of the impact of appearances in any organization. The compliance professional needs clout to get the job done,[14] and to deter efforts to undercut the compliance function. There must thus be a consideration of the signs and trappings of power.

In internal organizational politics, two signs of power are one's pay and one's title. In the compliance field there is occasionally the tendency to appoint a compliance "officer" who is really a mid-level manager with very little real authority. This person is rarely entitled to participate in senior management meetings as one of the decision makers. If a company claims that its compliance officer is a high-level person, then it is fair to ask what the person's salary is. Unless it is in the range of other senior officers, a skeptical observer could conclude that the company is more interested in the appearance of commitment, but is not fully prepared to put its cash behind its statements of commitment.

In a similar vein, fellow employees will assess the physical facilities, including offices and other perks, to gauge the real power and ranking of the compliance officer and staff. Availability of support staff is also a key element. If the compliance professionals lack the human resources to get the job done, this sends the signal that their work is not really a priority in the company.

Some companies have attempted to address the issues covered in this discussion by selecting as the compliance officer someone perceived as an "elder statesperson," close to retirement. The belief is that this person will be freer to express opinions and will be less easy to intimidate. Such a person will have the advantage of familiarity with the industry and the company's operations and personnel.

A countervailing school of thought challenges this approach, and would position the compliance function as a more active role, even as a path to promotion. From this perspective, there is concern about relying on an elder statesperson approach. If the designated person is in "senior" status, there may still be risk to the person's pension and other retirement benefits. There is also the risk that other key managers may more easily marginalize the person who is seen as being at the end of a career. It may be easier just to ignore this temporary compliance person who will soon be retiring from the company. Relying on the senior person also raises questions about the status of the staff who depend on the compliance officer for ongoing support for their activities. Just like the compliance officer whose primary protection is a golden parachute, when the compliance officer "bails out," the rest of the staff is left to deal with the same difficult issues.

If compliance staff are willing to step headlong into controversy, then they may be ready to address the next issue relating to power and protection—the ability to have input into the objectives and evaluations of others in the company.[15] If the compliance officer has a say in how other managers are appraised, this is certainly a sign of significant influence in the company. This process could start with the setting of officers' objectives for the year. Input from the compliance officer could ensure that compliance and ethics will be on the agendas of all the other officers and their departments. When the annual appraisals occur, the compliance officer would have direct input into the assessment of these other managers. If an officer was noted for dragging his or her heels on having employees trained or failing to follow up on findings from compliance audits, then that officer would see the negative impact in pay and in the ability to be promoted. As part of this same process, the compliance office could also review all promotions.

Although protecting the senior-most compliance official is key for the compliance program, there is also the issue of the subordinate managers whose work is essential to the success of the program. Protection of the compliance officer is not necessarily the same as protection of this staff. For example, the compliance officer may have a rich buy-out arrangement, but if the officer avails him- or herself of this tool, then it does nothing to protect others working in the program.

What are the options for protecting the staff? A number of the steps already covered are most practical for this purpose. If the company is willing to enter into an employment contract with the compliance officer, then the same step can be considered for the subordinate personnel. Similarly, if the board directs that it alone may make decisions about the tenure of the compliance officer, then it may also want to require that decisions about subordinate personnel at least be brought to the board's attention at some stage in the process. The issue of direct access to assistance and authority also comes into play here. Consideration can be given to providing access for subordinate compliance professionals with respect to the legal department, internal audit, the audit committee, and other key resources. This may be particularly appropriate when the company has a high-level compliance officer with many other responsibilities who delegates real compliance responsibility to an assistant compliance officer. In those cases especially there is great value in giving this person direct access to important power positions in the company.

Additional considerations apply when companies have separate business units with their own compliance staff. A subsidiary unit may have its own compliance officer, director, or coordinator. These business unit compliance program managers are valuable to the overall program because they help bring the compliance program into the field. To have the maximum impact, these managers need to be trusted by the other business unit managers, including the senior managers, and be close to all that is happening in that unit.

This, of course, raises the risk that such a person, operating separately from the corporate staff, may feel cut off from the mainstream of the company's compliance program and more vulnerable to the demands of local management. Ensuring that they have the requisite degree of independence and freedom from interference can require a strong connection with the headquarters compliance office. One of the key elements in protecting this status is to ensure that the business unit compliance staff members have direct, unfiltered access to the headquarters staff and the compliance office. Never can it be acceptable for anyone in the business unit to require that all such communications first be cleared or channeled through someone else. A second key element is to ensure that the compliance officer or the headquarters compliance staff has control of, or at least strong input into, the objectives, assessment, and advancement decisions affecting the business unit compliance personnel.

THE ROLE OF THE PROFESSION

Thus far the focus has been what the individual compliance professional and the specific company can do to strengthen and protect the professional. This is a substantial challenge and one that is especially difficult to accomplish in isolation. Moreover, whatever the individual professional may achieve in his or her own backyard, there is always the risk that an aggressive regulator or a judge unfamiliar with compliance activity will completely undercut the compliance function. If one regulator or jury seizes on a company's compliance activities to exploit these in a way that makes the company look foolish, the compliance professional's credibility and effectiveness can be mortally wounded.

It is in this context of a hostile legal system and a politically hazardous working environment that the issue of the role of professionalism comes into play. How does the acceptance of compliance as a true profession affect the compliance professional?

One characteristic of professionalism is the existence of a set of ethical standards that guide the professional. If compliance professionals are guided by such a set of ethical standards, these can add stature to the role that they play. Setting standards that mandate a high caliber of conduct can help empower the compliance professional. With strong, enforceable standards, the professional can use these ethical rules as a means for fending off suggestions or even strong pressure to engage in improper conduct.

Ethical standards help establish a measurement reference that is outside of the employer's pay standards.

Professional standards can help gain respect for the compliance professional and, as a result, compliance programs in general. Judges and prosecutors, who are themselves professionals, can more easily identify with those who are held to high, externally imposed standards of behavior. This can lend a welcome element of credibility to the compliance professional whose tasks may well include being asked to testify in support of an employer's efforts to receive lenient treatment because it had instituted an effective and credible program. Although all professions, because they consist of human beings, have their share of disreputable characters, it is possible to draw from the examples of attorneys and auditors as two groups whose professional standards are given weight and accepted within and outside of their employing organizations.

An organized profession has much more to offer than a set of professional standards, as valuable as that resource can be. The organization can be crucial in gaining legislative and political recognition where this is needed. A professional organization should be an active public voice for the profession. An example of where this would come into play can be seen in the flap in the United States about the application of the Fair Credit Reporting Act (FCRA) to companies that hire outside experts to conduct internal compliance investigations in response to allegations of misconduct.[16]

In April 1999, a Federal Trade Commission (FTC) staff attorney issued an opinion that in-house managers needed to get the *permission* of any employee targeted by an allegation of wrongdoing before hiring someone outside to conduct the investigation. To complete the absurdity, the opinion also stated that once a report was received from this outside firm, a full copy of the report had to be given to the person who was investigated. Thus, if a hospital had a serious allegation that one employee was causing harm to patients, and it hired an outside national law firm to conduct the investigation, before hiring the outside firm it would have to get the permission of the target of the allegation. When the confidential detailed opinion of outside counsel was then received, it would have to be given in its entirety to the target of the investigation, even if the report listed confidential sources, and even if the target were guilty beyond peradventure of the offenses. The lessons of the FCRA example were that no one at the FTC truly understood compliance, and that the compliance professionals did not have an organized voice to protest such misguided policy adventures.

In fact, it was other federal agencies that had to point out to the FTC how misguided this interpretation was.

An organized profession can also provide important support for the compliance professional. It can arrange training, resources, sources of guidance, and other assistance. The profession also has an enormous potential role in helping increase the recognition of effective compliance programs. It can put voice to the nature of this work, articulate how difficult this mission is, and demonstrate how compliance professionals help to protect not just their employers but society in general.

Performing the compliance mission in-house can sometimes lead to challenges to one's judgment, and to organizational resistance that can wear down an ordinary person. An organized compliance profession can facilitate access to and networking with compliance peers at other organizations. Whether through formal congresses of compliance professionals, or through the informal networking that the profession can foster, professionals are provided the ability to compare their treatment to the treatment of peers at other companies. It also allows for benchmarking, so that professionals can gain from the experiences of their peers elsewhere. As participants have noted about compliance practices forums, these contacts provide personal validation and support.[17]

Finally, the networking and access with peers give professionals another source of strength, namely, knowledge of the employment scene outside of the corporate walls. It is noble to ask compliance professionals to be prepared to fight wrongdoing, and to be prepared to leave the walls of the corporate campus if management persists in pursuing misconduct. But if the professional has a solid sense of where the next paycheck may come from, then it may be easier to take risky internal steps to deter wrongdoing.

The compliance professional, when joined by colleagues in the profession, can work within the existing system to maximize the strength and durability of the compliance role. But there also needs to be attention given to whether that existing system is enough, or whether compliance professionals should be pushing for changes to increase the effectiveness of compliance staff, and of compliance programs in general. Should the organized profession seek resort to the political and legal arena? If so, what types of protection should be pursued?

One option to consider would be a form of individual immunity for compliance professionals who perform compliance work in good faith. Membership in an organized profession that adhered to professional standards could be set as the price for gaining such protection. Those who adhered to such standards could be granted some degree of insulation from the "slings and arrows" of the legal process. The premises for such protection could be analogous to the state statutes that provide tort immunity for companies who discipline employees for misconduct, and then communicate the basis for that action to the employee body so that they all learn from the experience.[18] Another possibility would be a form of whistleblower protection for compliance professionals. This may be a less attractive approach, because it would pit the compliance professionals against their employers, by giving the employee the right to sue the employer.

In the governmental and political front, it is worth noting that the government also has a key leadership role to consider. In a very real sense, the compliance program and its professionals are doing the government's work for it. White-collar crime prevention and detection has, to a significant extent, been going through the process of privatization. Government initiatives, such as the Sentencing Guidelines, the Occupational Safety and Health Administration (OSHA) Voluntary Protection Program, and the Antitrust Division's Corporate Leniency Program, have offered substantial rewards to companies that join the law enforcement partnership.[19] The more government agencies and courts take this step, the more likely it is that companies will adopt real, not paper, programs, and the more likely it is that the compliance professionals who are placed in harm's way will have the tools and authority they need to do their jobs effectively. If, for example, the Department of Health and Human Services (HHS) were to recognize the importance of the compliance professional and the enormous significance that professional standards have in enhancing the credibility of compliance programs, the ability of these front-line soldiers to hold their positions and bring success to the war against white-collar crime and misconduct would be greatly enhanced.

CONCLUSION

The compliance function, like any management function, needs strong leadership and able implementation. Unlike most other management functions, however, it brings to the corporate table a mission not directly bent to the will of the organization. It exists to protect the company, but also to protect society and the values society considers important enough to make into laws. It may be true that companies benefit in the long term from taking the high road, but this perspective does not protect the compliance professional who may be the only one willing to raise a voice in dissent against a profitable but improper course of action.

To be effective in the business world, compliance officers who run these programs need the authority or, as the Australians label it, the clout to get the job done. For these programs to work effectively they also need effective, highly placed managers seeing to it that the programs work as designed in the rough and tumble of the business world. Yet, an intelligent manager will quickly see the downsides and risks to this type of pursuit. To keep good people doing this valuable work, they need support and protection. They should have the recognition and support that enables them to achieve their difficult goals.

This environment calls for the compliance professional to be alert to the risks, and also to have the means to reduce those risks. The message to the compliance professional is this: if you tend only your own compliance garden, you may well end up with bitter fruits. As a compliance professional you need to make sure you have the power and protection to do the job. You cannot afford to depend on someone else's largesse to get this for you. Whether it is working within the company, or joining with other compliance professionals to get the necessary external reforms, you can make the difference and make the job of the compliance professional a pursuit that benefits you, your company, and the society.

NOTES

1. *See* Chapter 3, *A Model for the Compliance Professional: Consulting, Policing, and Managing.*

2. *See* J. Murphy, *Examining the Legal and Business Risks of Compliance Programs*, 13 ETHIKOS 1 (Jan/Feb 2000).

3. See the list of functions set forth in the Sentencing Guidelines, U.S. SENTENCING GUIDELINES MANUAL § 8A1.2, comment (n 3(k)) (1993).

4. *See* J.M. KAPLAN ET AL., COMPLIANCE PROGRAMS AND THE CORPORATE SENTENCING GUIDELINES 6:17–6:19 (1993 & Ann. Supp.).

5. Under Kolstad v. American Dental Ass'n, 527 U.S. 526 (1999), for example, compliance efforts would be a defense to punitive damages in an employment discrimination case.

6. For examples of business attorneys being prosecuted for alleged involvement in business misconduct, see Bennett & Kris, *Under the Microscope: Business Lawyers are being Probed as Never Before*, 9 BUS. L. TODAY 10 (May/June 2000).

7. *See* J.M. KAPLAN ET AL., COMPLIANCE PROGRAMS AND THE CORPORATE SENTENCING GUIDELINES § 13:22 (1993 & Ann. Supp.).

8. Pearce v. E.F. Hutton Group, Inc., 664 F. Supp. 1490 (D.D.C. 1987).

9. E. Schultz, *Employees Beware: The Boss May Be Listening*, WALL STREET JOURNAL, July 29, 1994, at C1.

10. In re Caremark Int'l Inc. Derivative Litigation, 689 A.2d 959 (Del. Ch. 1996).

11. J. Braithwaite & J. Murphy, *Clout and Internal Compliance Systems*, 2 CORP. CONDUCT Q. 52–53 (1993).

12. For a more extensive discussion of compliance officer employment contracts, see J.E. Murphy, *Enhancing the Compliance Officer's Authority: Preparing an Employment Contract*, 11 ETHIKOS 5 (May/June 1998).

13. *See* N. Roberts, *Antitrust Compliance Programs under the Guidelines: Initial Observations from the Government's Viewpoint*, 2 CORP. CONDUCT Q. 1–3 (1992).

14. J. Braithwaite & J. Murphy, *Clout and Internal Compliance Systems*, 2 CORP. CONDUCT Q. 52 (1993).

15. Although the Sentencing Guidelines omit reference to evaluations and assessments as part of a compliance program, the OIG Guidance documents do lay the groundwork for input by compliance staff. *See, e.g.*, DEPARTMENT OF HEALTH AND HUMAN SERVICES, OFFICE OF INSPECTOR GENERAL, COMPLIANCE PROGRAM GUIDANCE FOR CLINICAL LABORATORIES, § II A 9, Compliance as an Element of a Performance Plan (Aug. 24, 1998).

16. *See* B. Yannett & L. Schachter, *FTC Applies FCRA to Firms*, NAT'L L.J. C1 (Feb. 14, 2000).

17. A. Gill, *Telecommunications Industry Practice Forum, in* UNITED STATES SENTENCING COMMISSION, CORPORATE CRIME IN AMERICA: STRENGTHENING THE "GOOD CITIZEN" CORPORATION, Proceedings of the Second Symposium on Crime and Punishment in the United States 89–90 (Sept. 7–8, 1995, Washington, DC).

18. *See, e.g.*, Merlo v. United Way, 43 F.3d 96, 103–05 (3d Cir. 1994). (Publication of an internal investigation report at a press conference protected under Florida and Virginia law.)

19. HHS has made statements promoting voluntary compliance programs, but has lagged behind other agencies that have been willing to make commitments of benefits to those either who have such programs or who step forward to disclose violations voluntarily.

Resolution Adopting a Compliance Program

WHEREAS, this Corporation has, from its beginning, been committed to integrity and responsible conduct, and to service to its community; and

WHEREAS, this Corporation is committed to conduct itself with the highest integrity and in compliance with all laws, and to help its members to understand the requirements of those laws that apply to the Corporation; and

WHEREAS, the Corporation has been assessing and enhancing its efforts to ensure adherence to these principles, and wishes to consolidate these efforts into one program;

NOW, THEREFORE, BE IT RESOLVED, that this Board hereby endorses those efforts and adopts as the highest policy of this Corporation, in the United States and abroad, a diligent ethics and compliance program (the Ethics and Compliance Program), under the direction of a Compliance Officer to be elected by this Board; and

BE IT FURTHER RESOLVED, that it is the policy of the Corporation to be a good citizen corporation, to cooperate in government investigations of wrongdoing, to make appropriate voluntary self-disclosures of violations of law, as determined by the Compliance Officer with the advice of the General Counsel, and to remedy any harm caused by such wrongdoing; and

BE IT FURTHER RESOLVED, that the Board hereby delegates to the Audit Committee of this Board responsibility for oversight of the Ethics and Compliance Program including participation in the annual evaluation of, and setting of compensation and incentives for, the Compliance Officer, and the Audit Committee shall give a detailed, annual report to the Board on the progress of the Program and plans for its future activities; and

---

Source: Copyright © Joseph E. Murphy.

BE IT FURTHER RESOLVED, that _____ is hereby elected as the Compliance Officer for this Corporation, to serve in that position until a successor is elected by this Board. The Compliance Officer, as an executive officer of this Corporation, shall have the authority and responsibility to take all appropriate steps deemed reasonably necessary for the establishment and operation of the Ethics and Compliance Program, including:

1. Working with all members of the Corporation to establish a program that is diligent, meets or exceeds industry practice, fosters the highest ethical standards, is effective in preventing and detecting violations of law, and meets or exceeds government standards including those set forth in the United States Sentencing Commission's Organizational Sentencing Guidelines;
2. Delegating to others in the Corporation responsibility for assisting in implementing the Ethics and Compliance Program;
3. Providing a detailed report on the Ethics and Compliance Program at each meeting of the Audit Committee, including training, discipline, development of standards and procedures, compliance auditing and monitoring, changes in compliance program personnel, reports of misconduct received through the reporting system, the handling of conflicts of interest, and any government investigations that may involve the Corporation; and
4. Informing the Chairman of the Audit Committee of any allegations of misconduct involving any senior official of the Corporation, prior to the disposition of any such allegation, and any instance when a recommendation of the Compliance Officer has been rejected or not followed; and

BE IT FURTHER RESOLVED that all actions previously taken by any officer or director of the Corporation prior to the date of these resolutions in connection with the actions contemplated by these resolutions are hereby ratified, confirmed, and approved in all respects; and

BE IT FURTHER RESOLVED, that the ongoing success of the Ethics and Compliance Program, and the Corporation's commitment to ethical conduct, is the personal responsibility of each manager and employee of the Corporation, and no other objective shall have a higher priority.

Employment Contracts for Compliance Officers: A Checklist

The following is a checklist of items to consider in preparing an employment contract for a compliance officer ("CO"), assistant compliance officer, or other compliance professional. It may not be necessary or possible to obtain coverage of each of these items in every contract, but they do raise points to be considered in the process of empowering a compliance manager.

1. Recitation of company's commitment to integrity and compliance, and to having a program at least as good as the Sentencing Guidelines and industry practice. Recite specifically that the company intends the program to be a "best practices" program, if that is the case. Contract to be construed in light of that commitment.
2. Description of position and job requirements: to ensure execution of the board's resolution committing the company to implement the ethics/compliance program. Such a resolution should be adopted.
3. Recitation that CO must conduct self with highest integrity, and conform to HCCA Code of Ethics for Health Care Compliance Professionals.
4. CO's position to be a "senior officer," consistent with definition in the Sentencing Guidelines. Specify the title, for example, Chief compliance and ethics officer, etc.

Source: Adapted with permission from J. Murphy, Enhancing the Compliance Officer's Authority: Preparing an Employment Contract, 11 *ethikos* 5 (May/June 1998).

5. CO to report to CEO and to audit committee (or other committee of outside directors) of the board. CO to have unrestricted access to the board committee.
6. Compensation and other incentives to be commensurate with senior officer status. Try to avoid connection of compensation to activities CO is expected to monitor. For example, it is better to tie incentives to long-term stock performance than to annual sales.
7. Specify who is to conduct CO's evaluation. Role of audit committee in this process.
8. Provide for length of term, to protect CO's position. Renewable on what terms.
9. Decision to renew to be made by audit committee, with advice of management. If decision is made not to renew, must be a written explanation by the audit committee.
10. The CO may be terminated for cause, upon the recommendation of the audit committee, and the vote of the whole board of directors.
11. Cause justifying termination of the CO means (a) a criminal act, or an act of moral turpitude, dishonesty, theft, unethical business conduct; (b) refusal to obey lawful orders given by the audit committee; or (c) failure to perform the responsibilities of this contract, as determined by the audit committee.
12. Describe amount and nature of supporting staff, CO's ability to obtain appropriate staff (in terms of numbers and quality), and CO's degree of control over that staff.
13. CO to have appropriate budget and resources.
14. CO to have direct access to company counsel. Recite that counsel represents company, and CO's discussions with counsel may be disclosed by counsel only to audit committee.
15. CO to have ability to retain outside professionals and other experts, as necessary.
16. Arbitration of disputes. Possibly look to outside, knowledgeable source, such as the Ethics Officer Association.
17. To have same benefits as other senior officers.
18. Entitled to no less than ___ weeks vacation per year (or no less than other senior officers).
19. Status of office, facilities to be no less than "most favored vice president" in company. Location to be same as other senior officers.

20. CO to have unlimited access to facilities, records and personnel, and all senior management meetings.
21. CO not to be reassigned, transferred, demoted, or have additional duties added without written consent and prior notice to the audit committee.
22. The CO is subject to the company's code of conduct, unless the code imposes a requirement that is not legally mandated, and that would otherwise result in a violation of this agreement or the HCCA Code of Ethics.
23. CO is expected to keep current with industry practice and is encouraged to participate in professional, ethics and compliance associations, and to attend and give presentations at their meetings.
24. Nondisclosure provision, to have exception for CO to disclose to appropriate government agency prospective or past violations of law. Also, must disclose any conduct where disclosure is required by law.

CHAPTER 9

Organizational Ethics and Compliance

George Khushf

INTRODUCTION

Health care is in the midst of major structural changes. Among the more significant developments is the merging of mechanisms of payment and provision, most conspicuous in managed care arrangements, but present to different degrees everywhere. With this merger comes an overlap of administrative and clinical jurisdictions. In a real sense, organizations are now the agents of practice, not just individual physicians. As administrators and organizations take on new roles, an organizational ethic is needed to guide workers in the health care arena into these uncharted waters.

The compliance movement has arisen just as the need for an organizational ethic has become especially acute, and it promises to meet that need. However, in its present form, and as it is currently conceptualized, compliance cannot fulfill that promise. It is generally conceptualized too narrowly, as the assurance of behavior conforming to preestablished norms, and its current practice is governed more by existing power relations than it is by ethical norms. Further, no fruitful dialogue exists between those working in organizational ethics and those in compliance.

Although current forms of compliance cannot fulfill the needs associated with organizational ethics, this does not mean that a sharp line should be drawn between the two. There are two options at this stage: (1) those involved in developing compliance programs must expand their focus, in order to incorporate the concerns associated with an organizational ethic, or (2) they must appreciate the relative and limited role of compliance programs, and ask how those programs might be incorporated into a broader organizational ethic. Either approach demands a greater self-critical voice within the compliance movement. If genuine compliance professionals (rather than just compliance bureaucrats) are to emerge, then such a self-critical stance must become part of the activity of those involved in compliance programs. The self-critical voice is up to now absent, and the compliance movement is formed by the self-interest of compliance consultants working in collaboration with governmental agents, who now exercise their power in a disproportionate manner. Without the self-critical voice, compliance and organizational ethics should be regarded as antithetical, and health care institutions must struggle to advance organizational ethics in spite of their compliance programs. This chapter outlines (1) the need for an organizational ethic, (2) why compliance programs are insufficient, and (3) how a critical voice can and should be developed within the compliance movement, so that an appropriate form of professionalism emerges.

THE NEED FOR AN ORGANIZATIONAL ETHIC

The Classical Biomedical Model: Organizations as "Silent Players"

The United States has long had a fee-for-service, indemnity-based system of health care. Within this system, an insured patient goes to a physician for care. The two jointly determine what is needed. When the transaction is complete, any needed tests or services are submitted to the insurer, who reimburses costs.

A classical interpretation of the nature of medicine is presupposed by this system of insurance. Following George Engel, this classical interpretation will be termed the "biomedical model."[1] It has the following components. First, it is assumed that the physician has an independent, natural scientific basis for determining what tests and services are indicated. When a patient comes to a physician with a health care need, that physician acts like a research scientist. From the symptoms discovered through the patient's history and the signs found in the initial physical exam, a physician constructs a disease hypothesis that is then confirmed, ruled out, or revised by laboratory tests. Where such tests are unavailable, the effective management of the patient's condition is regarded as a probabilistic confirmation of the disease hypothesis. What the physician does or does not do thus depends on the scientific method, not on any variable values or economic incentives. It is also assumed that the patient's need can be addressed piecemeal. The diagnosis and treatment of illness is divisible into parts, which can be addressed by individual tests, office visits, and procedures. This first assumption is referred to as the atomistic, scientifically foundational character of biomedicine.[2]

Second, it is assumed that the primary ethical responsibility of a physician is to the individual patient, not a community or patient population.[3] Professional ethics focuses on so-called micro-ethics; namely, the ethics of an individual–individual relation. The physician–patient interaction is a fiduciary relation. The patient is vulnerable as a result of sickness, and at a disadvantage because of asymmetrical power and knowledge. The physician is to act as an agent on the patient's behalf, ensuring that his or her best interest is protected. This second assumption, with its focus on the physician–patient relation and individual patient interest, is referred to as the micro-ethic of biomedicine.

Third, it is assumed that financial considerations should come into play at only the end, after the "medically indicated" course of treatment has been provided to the patient.[4] Health care is thus understood as a two-step process. First is the physician–patient relation and the practice of good medicine. Then, second, invoices for any costs incurred are submitted to an insurer for reimbursement. The clinical ethics of the physician–patient relation is thus neatly separable from the business ethics of the insurer or governmental systems of payment; micro-ethics is neatly separable from macro-ethics. This third assumption is referred to as the disjunct between clinical practice and economic considerations. This, in turn, leads to a disjunct between clinical and business ethics.[5]

These three assumptions have worked together with the fee-for-service, indemnity-based systems of insurance. The atomistic, scientifically foundational character of medicine justified approaching medicine in terms of billable pieces, each part determined independently and submitted for reimbursement. Insurers were separate from providers, and they traditionally exercised no authority over what was done or how medicine was practiced. Organizations were not regarded as agents of care. Either they provided the locus of practice (the hospital) or they reimbursed costs (the insurer). But their appropriate role was as a "silent player," never intruding into the matters of clinical care, which was the province of the physician.[6] According to the classical, biomedical model, any intrusion of social or economic values into the clinical decision-making process would involve a violation of both the scientific and ethical integrity of medicine.

A New Role for Organizations as Agents of Care

One of the most conspicuous developments in health care today involves the emergence of organizations as active agents of care.[7] The key question is how to assess this new role; whether to see it as something positive or negative. Consider the following areas where institutions and administrators now encroach upon the clinical domain:[8]

- *The designation of generalists as gatekeepers.* Some health plans require that patients always first see a generalist, who provides primary care and only refers when a referral is clearly indicated. The physician gatekeeper usually serves two functions: (1) to ensure that the best kind of care is provided and (2) to reduce the costs associated with care, especially specialist care. Sometimes these functions can conflict.
- *The establishment of a hospital formulary.* At many health care institutions a pharmacist, usually in consultation with physicians, will give priority to certain drugs over others. A physician who seeks to use an alternative drug in the same class is then required to justify that usage. Because the separate justification may require additional time and effort on the part of the physician, it is more likely that the default drug will be chosen. In addition to standardizing the drug regimen, the purpose of such a formulary is to control costs, because a hospital can obtain discounts on the drugs when it gives them priority. Some physicians believe that this compromises their capacity to provide the best clinical care.
- *The provision of financial incentives for reduced utilization of services.* These financial incentives may come in several forms. An insurer may provide bonus and withholding arrangements for physicians, so that physicians obtain additional income if they demonstrate a pattern of utilization that involves lower costs. In other cases, physicians or a physician group practice (perhaps owned by a hospital) may receive a capitated payment for a group of patients. Physicians must then provide services to this group. Often they must pay for certain basic tests out of the pool of funds obtained by the capitated payments. As a result they have a strong financial incentive to reduce the services that they provide for patients.

In each of these cases, an insurer or hospital influences how health care is practiced. An administrative and organizational interest in stewardship of resources is passed on to physicians in such a way that the standard of clinical care is directly altered.

Although much of the literature on such developments focuses upon the economic incentives, these are not the only ones that motivate this "encroachment" of administrative influence. In the book, *Clinical Decision Making*, David Eddy outlines additional reasons why administrators are now challenging the physician's role as decision maker.

> [W]hile the rapid and apparently uncontrollable rise in health care costs might have been the initial pressure point, the challenge can be justified solely by a concern for quality. The plain fact is that many decisions made by physicians appear to be arbitrary—highly variable, with no obvious explanation. The very disturbing implication is that this arbitrariness represents, for at least some patients, suboptimal or even harmful care.[9]

Among the developments in quality control, one finds the following kinds of strategies:

- *Guidelines and clinical pathways.* Institutions are now implementing guidelines. These are simplified rules for care, which maximize benefit over harm (and cost). The intent is to eliminate the variability associated with individualized decision making. Guidelines can be developed by professional organizations, but they come with different levels of sophistication. In all cases, they involve an attempt to codify the standard of care and incorporate information on outcomes of care so that unnecessary and ineffective care is not provided. Many physicians are concerned that such guidelines involve a "cook book medicine" that is insufficiently attentive to all of the nuances associated with medical decision making. Some guidelines now incorporate patient preferences and subjective assessments of quality, factors poorly understood and previously unaddressed. Eddy rightly notes that this involves a radical revision of the way the standard of care is formed within medicine.[10]
- *Attempts to eliminate medical mistakes.* Traditionally, medical mistakes have been understood as a problem of individuals, associated with people who do not practice according to a given standard of care, exhibiting either a failure of knowledge or a temporary lapse in judgment. When it is an individual problem, it is addressed in terms of

professional self-regulation. But today the problem of mistakes is increasingly configured as a systems problem, rather than an individual one, with the focus shifting to administrative policy for monitoring practice and ensuring accountability.[11] Institutions are thus assuming responsibility for addressing these matters of care.

- *The logistics of technology.* Institutions are no longer willing to serve as simply the locus for care, providing personnel and other resources to support the activity of physicians. They now recognize that much of care is technologically based, and that the logistics for coordinating these multimillion-dollar technology resources have a direct bearing on the care provided. In controlling this technology, they are increasingly controlling care. The care is now conceptualized as a team effort, involving multiple professionals who interact with patients, technology, and other professionals in a complex manner that is now coordinated by administrative oversight and policy.[12]

Whether associated with cost or quality, all of these developments pose a challenge to the traditional biomedical model, with its atomistic scientific foundationalism, individual patient orientation, and disjunct between clinical and economic considerations. The question is how this challenge can be best assessed. How does one evaluate the new, active role now played by organizations?

Within the extensive literature on recent developments in health care, one can identify two distinct responses.[13] The first sees the encroachment of administrative and organizational interests in negative terms, as a distortion motivated primarily by economic considerations that undermine the scientific and ethical core of modern medicine. Against this distortion, some attempt to reassert the older professional ideals and mitigate the influence of administrative authority. A strong distinction is sustained between clinical ethics and organizational ethics, with the latter understood as a form of business ethics.[14]

A second, more progressive response sees in these developments the emergence of a new form of health care. With this new form, however, there is a need to reassess the older ideals. Organizational ethics then involves a foundational, radical project; namely, the formulation of norms for a new paradigm of health care.[15] This chapter argues that this second, progressive approach is the appropriate one.

The Need for an Organizational Inter-Ethic

In the face of the current transformations taking place in health care, a neat distinction between micro- and macro-ethical domains can no longer be sustained. Institutions are not simply the loci of care or disinterested payers. As agents of care, they now exercise authority and are responsible for outcomes. This reality demands a thorough rethinking of the assumptions found in the classical, biomedical model. Further, a new domain of ethical reflection for middle-level institutions is needed. One cannot view organizations as mini-states or as the mere concatenation of individual–individual relations. Until now, the needed inter-ethics, complementing the classical micro- and macro-ethics, has been absent.[16]

The rethinking of the role of organizations must be linked to a reassessment of the assumptions behind the biomedical model. This means, first, a critique of its atomistic, scientific foundationalism. This does not mean a move away from science, in order to embrace its opposite (although there are some developments that may be interpreted in this manner; for example, the increasing use of alternative and complementary medicines[17]). Rather, what is meant by "science" and how health care is conceptualized as scientific must be reconsidered.[18] In the past, the model of medicine as a science was drawn directly from the natural sciences. A physician was like a physicist calculating the trajectory of a projectile and then figuring out how to alter its course, although he or she had to use a probabilistic form of reasoning to handle uncertainty. Today it is apparent that other sciences, especially the human sciences, are just as much a part of medicine. In addition to pathoanatomy, pathophysiology, and the related biological, chemical, and physical sciences, health care draws on the psychological, social, and economic sciences. With the incorporation of subjective factors (for example, those associated with quality of life) into outcome assessments, the use of health services research for quality control, and the extensive utilization of systems engineering as a part of management, there is a more dialectical relation between the "facts" and "values" in medicine.[19] Further, and perhaps most significantly, a health problem cannot be broken into little pieces, so that each part is dealt with independent of the others. The web of care provided by organizations challenges the atomism of the traditional model. When one speaks of "medically necessary" care, one thus speaks of standards of care that are not just a function of the aggregate of decisions made by individual physicians.[20]

The clinical ethic of biomedicine also needs to be reassessed. If care is configured by organizations and depends on systemwide considerations, then it cannot be seen as just individually oriented. Care is also oriented toward communities, and strategies are developed that maximize the health of a population.[21] Ethical norms must thus address how to rightly balance the good of an individual against the good of a patient population.[22] This good of the population should not, however, be directly equated with the common good. An institution may be responsible for a population that is a small subset of the society; for example, a managed care plan responsible for those it insures. There will thus be a tension between individual and sub-population good, and also between sub-population good and the common good. An organizational ethic is needed to help work through how this subtle balancing between diverse interests is best approached.[23]

Just as there is a need for a new ethic for population-oriented health care, there is also a need for a new language for one that is organizationally based. If teams practice health care, not just individuals, how does one understand authority, responsibility, and accountability? So often patient care suffers because there is insufficient coordination between generalists, the multiple specialists that can be involved in a single case, nurse case managers, chaplains, social workers, and the multiple other professionals involved in care. The language of accountability at many institutions still presupposes that a patient has a single physician who is responsible for the care provided, and that the torch shifts from one to another and back again as the patient is transferred from unit to unit. There is no language for team accountability and an institutionally based practice. That must also come under the purview of an organizational ethic.

Finally, an organizational ethic is needed to work out how matters of provision and payment are integrated. Because the sharp disjunction between clinical and economic domains cannot be sustained, it must be asked how marginal utility is addressed in an equitable manner. These issues, traditionally under the purview of a macro-ethic, are now addressed in a pluralistic manner, and at the organizational level. This means that one institution may legitimately arrive at a different kind of balance—and thus a different standard of care—when compared with another institution.[24] There is not yet the ethical or legal apparatus for considering this organizationally based, pluralistic approach to the formation of a standard of care.

THE INSUFFICIENCY OF COMPLIANCE

The compliance movement arose in the midst of these radical changes in health care, and it promises to address problems in cost-control, quality, and ethics. Broadly understood, compliance is part of the federal government's war on waste, fraud, and abuse. The tools of the current war can be traced back to 1981, when section 1128A was added to the Social Security Act, authorizing the Secretary of Department of Health and Human Services (HHS) to impose civil monetary penalties (CMPs).[25] In 1993, health care reform efforts placed an emphasis upon the crisis in access and cost-control, and it was claimed that everyone could have everything as long as waste, fraud, and abuse were eradicated.[26] With this assumption, major efforts were launched to address the problem of waste, fraud, and abuse. The Secretary of HHS realigned the responsibility for enforcing CMPs, with the Health Care Financing Administration (HCFA) implementing those associated with program compliance, and the Office of Inspector General (OIG) implementing those associated with Medicare fraud. In August 1996, with the passage of the Health Insurance Portability and Accountability Act (HIPAA), CMPs up to $10,000 per item or service out of compliance, and up to treble the amount claimed, could be assessed.

In practice, the new fines could bankrupt nearly every health care institution, as all were out of compliance.[27] When these institutions recognized the potential liability, they passively accepted whatever was imposed upon them. So-called "voluntary" compliance guidelines were put forth by the OIG, and institutions were told that if they made a good-faith effort to implement them, then this would be taken into consideration when fines were assessed. Marks of a "good-faith effort" included how much money was spent on compliance programs and how independently and effectively these programs audited the behavior of those at the institution, with direct lines of reporting to the government agencies responsible for enforcement.[28] Effectively, health care institutions are now required to pay directly for extensive governmental mechanisms of monitoring and oversight, with hot lines from institution-paid informants directly to the governmental agencies. With an unprecedented power to destroy any health care institution that it chooses to bankrupt, institutions have been coerced to implement "ethics programs" patterned after the government's dictate.

Although there are significant problems with the way compliance programs have been imposed upon health care institutions, that is not the primary focus of these critical comments. The concern is rather with the ways those programs are deficient. Here the focus is on four problems. First, compliance programs have been insufficiently attentive to the clash between business considerations and professional ethics. Second, through a discussion of HCFA's proposed evaluation and management guidelines, it will then be shown how compliance initiatives presuppose exactly those elements of the biomedical model that are now called into question by recent developments in health care. Third, it will be shown that the notion of ethics in compliance is deficient. Finally, it will be shown that the notion of professionalism within the compliance movement is likewise deficient.

How Physicians View Their Obligations to Patients

In a classic study on truth-telling, published in the *Journal of the American Medical Association*, Novack et al. presented a case of a healthy, 52-year-old patient, Mrs. Lewis.[29] The physician wishes to order a screening mammogram, but discovers that it is not covered by the insurer. The patient is of modest means and cannot easily afford it. When told by his secretary that "the way to get around this is to put down 'rule out cancer' instead of 'screening mammography,'" the physician is asked which of the two should be put on the form. Among the 199 physicians who responded to the question, nearly 70 percent indicated that they would write "rule out cancer." In other words, 70 percent would commit fraud (although they would not view it as such).

In a more recent study, "Lying for Patients: Physician Deception of Third-Party Payers," Freeman et al. considered in detail physician attitudes toward insurers.[30] They provided realistic cases, drawn from the experiences of many physicians, and asked whether it was legitimate to use deception. The conclusion fully confirmed the results of the earlier study: "Many physicians sanction the use of deception to secure third-party payers' approval of medically indicated care."[31] What is most interesting is that physicians view such deception as *ethically* warranted when systems of payment indicate basic irrationalities; for example, when the rules prevent payment for services that are in some cases clearly life-saving.[32] One essay, in summarizing this study, highlights the clash between two loyalties. "The dilemma is between acting as the patient's agent . . . or violating the trust of the third-party payer."[33] Daniel Sulmasy, one of the investigators, "said his findings on physician willingness to use deception to secure coverage indicated a broader societal problem. 'Why is it that we have a system of health care that puts physicians in this impossible dilemma?'"[34]

These studies are not cited to claim that the current willingness of physicians to defraud insurers is appropriate, or that this willingness indicates a high standard of professionalism. To the contrary, this behavior needs to be changed, compliance can play an important role in that change, and there is an overlap between efforts to alter such behavior and broader initiatives associated with medical professionalism.[35] But the current tension between a clinical ethic that emphasizes fiduciary obligations and the business ethic of compliance needs to be seriously addressed, and the deficiencies in current mechanisms of financing must be discussed. As Sulmasy notes, there are broader societal problems that lie behind issues of billing. Within the bioethical arena, there is an extensive literature on these problems and the possible resources for working through them ethically. However, those in the compliance arena speak as if the problem is simply one of compliance or its lack. At a plenary session of a Health Care Compliance Association meeting (Region IV, April 28–30, 1999, in Atlanta, Georgia), I asked Jim Sheehan, one of the primary architects of compliance initiatives, about these problems. His answer was indicative: "I'm sorry. I see these matters in terms of black and white. Either you obey the law or you don't." Surely we need a more nuanced answer than that. Behind the clash between professional ethics and compliance, there are deeper issues of organizational ethics; for example, issues associated with integrating patient best interest with a broader institutional and social accountability. Physicians are struggling with how to sustain trust and professionalism in the face of forces that seem to undermine these. Their willingness to use deceit highlights a helplessness that needs to be addressed as a part of the very compliance efforts that counter that deceit. Unfortunately, all compliance gives is a notion of ethics that emphasizes conformity to pre-established rules, whether or not those rules are appropriate, and whether or not a patient will die as a result. This only breeds cynicism with respect to the process of compliance and undermines its legitimacy.

A Case Study: The Evaluation and Management Guidelines

One of the best studies of compliance to date has been provided by Allan Brett in an essay for the *New England Journal of Medicine* titled "New Guidelines for Coding Physician's Services—A Step Backward."[36] Although Brett focuses his attention on the evaluation and management services, his criticisms apply more generally to all of compliance. His study can thus be taken as a good review of the deficiencies associated with the implicit assumptions of compliance. At the risk of altering his emphasis somewhat, Brett's arguments are summarized here according the three assumptions of biomedicine outlined earlier.

First, consider the atomistic foundationalism of biomedicine. Brett notes that:

> HCFA has patterned the guidelines on a particular conception of clinical reasoning. According to that conception, the clinical encounter is essentially a compilation of bits of history and pieces of physical examination; the complexity of the encounter is roughly proportional to the numbers of bits and pieces.[37]

The physician is supposed to count elements of medical, family, and social history; count organ systems and body areas reviewed; and tally the kinds of physical examination associated with each organ system. Then the different parts are incorporated into a table with an assessment of potential complications, and, after some complex combinations, come up with the appropriate code. After reviewing the process, Brett concludes that "this attempt to capture clinical reasoning is too linear," missing the subtle way hypotheses are actually developed and refined.

Brett is especially concerned about the impact of these assumptions— and the coding requirements—on patient care, noting that "the trends in documentation and coding embodied by the evolving HCFA guidelines violate the ethical principle of providing care that is in the best interests of patients."[38] Note how the second assumption, that of an individual patient focus, comes into his analysis. By requiring that the patient's chart be cluttered with information that is not of use in patient care, and by diverting a significant amount of the physician's time to administrative and billing considerations, the usefulness of the chart and time for patient care is diminished. Further, the patterns used for coding distort the clinical reasoning process itself.

This last point brings Brett to the third assumption of biomedicine; namely, the disjunct between clinical practice and economic considerations. In response to those who contend that billing considerations should simply come in as a second step, after the appropriate medical care has been provided to the patient, he notes:

[T]his assumption is naive. Coding guidelines influence the substance of the clinical encounter, because they implicitly specify the elements of a medical encounter that are valued by those who compensate physicians for their work.[39]

Physicians are taught how to bill and thereby learn to configure their practice so that fair compensation is obtained. Without question, financial incentives influence practice. This fact is at the heart of the incentive structures found in managed care, and it is well documented by empirical studies. To assume the opposite involves ignoring nearly everything in the health services research literature.

This brief review has not done justice to the depth of Brett's analysis. The intent here has been to simply highlight some of his conclusions, and indicate the kind of critical analysis that should be associated with compliance efforts at all levels. Unfortunately, this kind of foundational criticism has been almost completely absent within the Health Care Compliance Association (HCCA) and among the governmental agents and consultants involved in the movement. If compliance is to be developed appropriately, just those outside must not level the criticism. It must be incorporated as an essential activity of the compliance professional. In fact, such a critical development can be regarded as continuous with compliance itself. After all, compliance efforts are now directed toward certain financial arrangements such as managed care, which are at risk of diminishing quality. Why not take the next step and ask about the influence of compliance programs themselves? What is their impact on quality? What financial, quality, and ethical risks are posed by compliance programs?

A Deficient Approach to Ethics

In the bioethics and compliance literature there are two very different understandings of the nature of ethical reflection. In bioethics literature, "ethics" has a nuanced and rich meaning, involving a complex confluence of moral and religious traditions, social policy, culture, and law. In compliance, by contrast, ethics is understood narrowly, as behavior conforming to previously articulated norms. The compliance definition is truncated and becomes problematic in contexts where the norms are or should be changing.

To best understand the way ethics is conceptualized in the bioethics literature, it is helpful to briefly provide a historical overview of the emergence of the field.[40] Although a medical professional ethic is ancient, hearkening back at least to the Hippocratic tradition, bioethics as a field is a relatively recent phenomenon. Like compliance, it emerged in the context of radical ferment and change. The legal background of the field was set against the civil rights movement, and a series of legal cases that challenged the hegemony of medical decision making and values in the context of patient care. In addition to prominent cases associated with informed consent, there were also celebrated cases on the withholding and withdrawing of care. The most celebrated case here was that of Karen Ann Quinlan, a patient in a vegetative state on a respirator. The family wanted withdrawal of this aggressive care, something resisted by the health care providers involved with the case.

This case, and many of the developments associated with the rise of bioethics as a field, would not be understandable without the amazing technological developments in medicine that emerged in the last three decades. Although there were longstanding precedents on withholding and withdrawing care (especially in the Catholic tradition), physicians did not previously have the capacity to keep people alive with machines, people who otherwise would have been long dead. Increasingly it was asked: Just because something can be done, does that mean that it should be done? This was the kind of question that outsiders started asking—theologians, philosophers, attorneys, and family members, among others—and the rise of bioethics is directly linked to this shift from a traditional medical professional ethic toward a broader ethical and social configuration of the problems.

Although law played a significant role in this development, it was not the only or even the primary influence. Consider, for example, the so-called "God squad" in Seattle, which was responsible for allocating scarce resources available for dialysis. When physicians involved in patient care were faced with deciding who lives and who dies, they recognized that they needed outside help in making these decisions. The committee responsible for addressing this concern included prominent philosophers and theologians, who addressed the questions of equitable distribution. There was broad critical reflection on how new developments in health care could be best addressed, and a consensus gradually emerged on what was appropriate; for example, that one should not utilize social worth criteria in making those decisions.

Another development in clinical bioethics was almost completely separate from law. As problems in withholding end-of-life care moved from being a rare exception to a regular feature of modern medicine, ethics committees formed at hospitals and other health care institutions.[41] Here the problem was not just what the law allowed; rather, given that it was legitimate to withhold or withdraw life-saving care, how was this to be addressed in individual cases? The model of ethics consultation was linked to a notion of "qualified facilitation," namely, through the consult a space independent of law and the standard hierarchies of medicine was opened up so that people could explore what the appropriate options were. The point of such ethics reflection was not simply to identify the law and then impose the rules; it was rather to provide the space for working through difficult cases where matters were not clearly black and white.

This last point is central. With health care changing so rapidly, there are many cases when the standard way of doing things just does not seem appropriate. Often those involved in a case will get just this awkward sense that something is wrong, but they cannot clearly articulate why they are uncomfortable. Here "ethics" is used to speak of a form of reflection, which steps back, critically evaluates the case in the light of deeper ethical principles involved, and then works toward an appropriate resolution. Standard ways of doing things—the implicit and explicit norms—may need to be revised. The skills involved in such deliberations are complex, and there has been a decade-long debate on how best to codify them, culminating in the recent report of the American Society for Bioethics and Humanities on the standards of ethics consultation.[42]

Summarizing, bioethics as a movement involves a rich coalescence of legal, theological, ethical, and social deliberation. It recognizes that rapid changes require a foundational, critical form of reflection, which reassesses the norms that have been taken for granted. Much of the efforts are associated with opening up a free space for continued deliberation and consensus formation. This is a difficult and relatively long process, and it has some clear deficiencies.[43] But in the long run, norms are articulated that are more attentive to the complexity of health care reality.

The contrast with compliance efforts could not be more obvious. Again radical developments in the health care arena are faced. A few of them have been outlined earlier in this chapter. In fact, within the bioethics arena, there have been efforts to think through some of these, especially under the rubric of organizational ethics, although these efforts are just in their germinal stage. However, with compliance there has been little open debate. Instead of addressing this through the common law tradition, with occasional legislative efforts associated with a codified consensus, compliance has come primarily from the government in a top-down manner. It does not appear that the legislature, when it contemplated the fines in the HIPAA, was or is aware of the kinds of disproportional power it was vesting upon the government. The potential liability to health care institutions is so great, and the initiative framed by a social and political climate so unconducive to careful deliberation, that nearly all health care institutions were forced to acquiesce to the "voluntary" ethics/compliance programs imposed.

One of the most problematic areas of compliance is associated with the way the language of ethics is used. No longer is it associated with the classical philosophical and theological traditions that have long informed ethical and legal analysis. Instead, it is given a very narrow meaning. Despite some language that attempts to qualify this, for all practical purposes "ethics" means conformity to law.[44] "Ethics officers,"[45] with very few exceptions, could not tell the difference between an act-based, consequence-oriented, or virtue ethic, nor could they provide even a cursory definition of words such as "right" or "good." They do not know anything about any of the moral traditions that have informed ethical analysis, and there is currently no attempt to incorporate such knowledge into their training or the certification programs associated with compliance. They have no skills whatsoever in working through the difficult issues of balancing individual and communal good, or navigating the complex issues of accountability in the new team contexts of health care.

Ethics officers are bureaucrats, not professionals. Corporate compliance officers are given a role at health care institutions analogous to the police. Although they may not see their role in this manner, this is clearly how it is seen by nearly all others in the health care arena. They are to educate people about policy, monitor behavior, and then bring sanction when a wrong (understood as a violation of the law) is identified. They are to set up their hotlines and negotiate their contracts so that there are no repercussions when they refer their cases to the appropriate law enforcement agencies involved. At best, they play only a marginal role in formulating the standards that are imposed by the government on health care institutions (and here, it is often the independent consultants, especially in smaller institutions with fewer resources for compliance), and, even when they have played this advisory role, those involved have little knowledge of the deeper ethical problems involved.

When ethics is framed in this way, there is a deleterious impact on virtue and ethics generally at institutions. People increasingly see the issues in terms of poorly developed laws and punishment, and many believe that the impact on quality of care at institutions will be harmed. Despite claims by the OIG to the contrary, there is little global assessment of the impact of compliance on quality. This, in fact, is one of the areas where critical reflection and research is greatly needed, but absent.

A Deficient Approach to Professionalism

Generally, there are two kinds of definitions of professionalism, one sociologically oriented, the other ethically oriented.[46] Both kinds acknowledge a base of knowledge or expertise and an autonomy for self-regulation. However, in the sociological literature, the emphasis is placed upon monopolistic power and the way this power can be used to advance the economic, political, and social prestige interests of the professional. This approach will be referred to here as the nonmoral approach to professionalism.[47] In the ethical definitions, by contrast, the emphasis is placed upon the social value of the profession and the moral fabric that binds professionals to advance a good that cannot otherwise be advanced.

As a movement, compliance is undoubtedly taking the steps needed to establish practitioners as professionals. It has established a Health Care Compliance Certification Board, and already has exams for certification.[48] A body of knowledge has been developed, and the organizations involved (primarily the HCCA) are positioning themselves to establish monopolistic control. The hope is that only certified compliance officers can serve in health care institutions. At conferences there is ample discussion about how contracts should be written to insulate them and their programs from the kinds of outside influences (for example, the medical professionals or hospital administrators) that might motivate them to allow standards that deviate from those codified within their body of knowledge and practice. One thus does find, at least in the first steps, a move for professionalism. Two questions, however, still need to be addressed. First, is there the kind of expertise and knowledge base that characterizes a genuine profession, or is it more akin to what one finds among bureaucrats? Second, is this movement motivated by economic gain and sociopolitical prestige, or, more appropriately, by a clearly articulated social good? Each of these will be considered in turn.

Put crudely, bureaucrats do not have a body of knowledge that has its own integrity. Instead, they are given their marching orders and goals by others, and then must find a way to realize these in a given setting. Professionals, by contrast, formulate their own goals, usually directed toward the realization of an important moral or social value, and then develop knowledge and expertise so that they realize these goals. Knowledge, and to a large extent, the goals themselves, are self-regulated. Given this distinction, it seems quite clear that those working in compliance do not have the body of knowledge that constitutes a genuine profession. They have received their norms and goals from the governmental agents that have imposed these "voluntary" programs on health care institutions. These external agents determine what is appropriate or inappropriate, not those in compliance. Once this is done, the norms for a strong compliance program are then passed on through the compliance consultants and others that configure the standards of practice.

Certainly there will be people who object to this contention. The leadership in HCCA and the influential consultants will point out that there has been an ongoing collaboration with the government, and they will claim that the standards have not come in a top-down manner, but rather have arisen out of this collaboration and under the guidance of those involved in compliance. However, the devil is in the details. Those who contend this should go through the formation of the guiding documents and initiatives, and in virtually every case there will be a clear asymmetry in the relations involved. Even bureaucrats can influence particular policies through their feedback. The key question is whether they, through their expertise, form the goals and knowledge base. The details of that formation cannot be delved into here, but debate on just this issue would be welcome, with the belief that the answer will be fairly clear. But even having debate on this would be a worthwhile first step. Not even that is present.

Now to the second question: Is this movement motivated by power, wealth, and prestige, or by a clearly articulated moral or social good? Before this question is answered, a clear distinction needs to be made between the majority of those who serve in compliance at health care institutions and the distinct minority involved in advancing the mechanisms of professionalization. There is little doubt that the majority of people involved and who attend compliance meetings and who are members in organizations such as the HCCA simply want to discover how to do their job well. Compliance guidelines have, for good or evil, been imposed on health care institutions and practitioners. As a result, people have been designated to address the compliance concerns, and they now work to address them in an appropriate manner. But this by itself does not explain the mechanisms of professionalization. And these mechanisms—namely, the certification boards, the high-priced consultation services, and the movement toward monopolistic practice—are a function of a select few, who have positioned themselves in ways that reinforce their power and control of the movement. Standards have not been forming in a democratic manner, from the grass roots upward, through a deliberative process. Instead, founding presidents move to be the presidents of new, subsidiary, or affiliated organizations. Officers and board members move from being head compliance officers to consultants, and these work with an inner circle that includes the key governmental agents at the pinnacle of power. Although this is a natural process, one would be hard pressed to see in the development an attempt to explore how compliance can best meet a given social need.

In sum: Compliance, defined as "meeting the expectation of others," is simply assumed as the appropriate end, with no question asked about whether the expectations are appropriate. Compliance officers are those who ensure conformity to expectation. The process of professionalism involves ensuring that these officers are well paid, protected, and given high regard. Although the motivation of most involved in the movement is simply to address their obligations in a competent manner, the motivation for professionalization, advanced by a minority of very influential consultants and leaders in the compliance movement, seems to be that of influence and power.

WHERE SHOULD WE GO FROM HERE? TOWARD A MORE APPROPRIATE FORM OF PROFESSIONALISM

The previous sections have shown that an organizational ethic is needed, and that there are significant deficiencies in the way compliance is understood and practiced. Unless compliance is reconfigured, so that it is responsive to the needs and realities of the current health care system, it should be seen as antithetical to organizational ethics. Compliance represents current constellations of power and must be addressed at health care institutions. But the task must be to minimize its harm, and advance an organizational ethic in spite of compliance programs. This will mean trying to recover the values that are generally undermined by current compliance efforts, especially in the areas of cultivating an appropriate notion of ethical reflection and advancing quality.

Thus far the comments made in this chapter have been framed in a very stark manner, perhaps too starkly. This has been intentional. It is the author's belief that there is little critical reflection within the movement, and it is hoped that this chapter will promote such reflection. That said, it is time to step back a little and frame some comments in a less critical manner. Many of the developments associated with compliance are greatly needed. The government has a legitimate interest in ensuring that people are not defrauded and that contractual obligations are fulfilled.[49] As any other payer, it has an interest in ensuring that it gets what it pays for (although it should not have an undue influence in this regard). The bioethics literature is likewise one-sided, needing many of the insights that are found within the compliance movement. Further, the kind of monitoring and accountability associated with compliance is simply one aspect of the radical development and transformation in health care outlined earlier. Compliance, together with other areas where organizations emerge as agents, is a phenomenon that calls for an appropriate organizational ethic. Compliance is here to stay. The question is now whether it can move to the next stage, and be transformed into a more appropriate form.

Although I am skeptical about the current trajectory of the compliance movement and also somewhat skeptical about whether this can be changed, there are some important counter-currents that could be intensified. Compliance need not be defined in such a narrow way. There are important moral and social values that could be featured as central within the movement, and a knowledge base could be formed, so that these values are appropriately addressed. A more open and deliberative process could be introduced, which mitigates the prestige and wealth interests that motivate the current process of professionalization. And there are valuable alliances that can be established with others who address similar problems, especially in the arenas of ethical deliberation associated with religious health care initiatives (for example, Catholic health systems) and bioethics. In closing, three areas where efforts are needed to expand the scope and function of compliance should be considered; namely, (1) the articulation of the values that direct compliance efforts, (2) an integration of compliance and organizational ethics, and (3) the development of a context open to research and critical reflection. These are the elements needed for a richer, moral notion of professionalism.

The Values that Direct Compliance

Within the HCCA, the value of compliance efforts is defined very narrowly, as the bureaucrat's concern of meeting others' expectations. However, within the OIG Guidelines, compliance is defined in a broader way, as advancing quality, ethics, and cost-control in the health care sector. As a first step, those involved in compliance should directly appropriate the values put forward by the OIG. However, if this is done, then a more critical process with respect to OIG Guidelines is needed.

The contrast between the HCCA values and those of the OIG can be well illustrated by a comparison of the HCCA Internet Homepage and a representative OIG Guideline (the guidance for hospitals will be taken as representative). On the HCCA Web site, compliance is defined narrowly as:

> The process of meeting the expectations of others. More specifically, it is the process of helping our health care professionals understand and meet the expectations of those who grant us money, pay for our services, regulate our industry, etc.[50]

The "Major Functions" of the organization are then defined as:

1. To promote quality compliance programs in health care—their introduction, development, and maintenance.
2. To provide a forum for interaction and information exchange to enable our members to provide high quality compliance programs.
3. To create high quality educational opportunities for those involved with compliance in the health care industry.

It is explicitly stated in bold letters and as a separate section:

HCCA is not meant to:

> Focus on clinical or bioethical compliance issues or duplicate the current efforts of general and specialty-specific national associations that lobby for regulatory changes.

In addition to the narrow, positive definition of compliance in terms of "meeting the expectations of others," note what is explicitly excluded. Compliance is strongly and explicitly separated from clinical and bioethical domains (although these remain undefined—what are the "bioethical compliance issues" that are excluded?), and it is to play no role in influencing the regulations that embody the expectations that compliance is supposed to meet. Further, nothing is said about an active domain of research and reflection, where compliance professionals work toward defining and articulating the norms of the discipline. Instead, it is assumed that those norms are formed by others—for example, by the consultants—and IICCA provides a forum where people can come and learn about these.

Now consider what the OIG Compliance Program Guidance for Hospitals says about compliance.[51] There it is assumed that, in addition to cost-control (a central concern behind the so-called "war on waste, fraud, and abuse"), compliance efforts directly advance quality and ethics. Three of many statements in this regard are cited here (the emphasis is added).

> The adoption and implementation of voluntary compliance programs significantly advance the prevention of fraud, abuse and waste in these health care plans while at the same time *furthering the fundamental mission of hospitals, which is to provide quality care to patients* (Section I).

> It is incumbent upon a hospital's corporate officers and managers *to provide ethical leadership to the organization and to assure that adequate systems are in place to facilitate ethical and legal conduct.* Indeed, many hospitals and hospital organizations have adopted mission statements articulating their commitment to high ethical standards. A formal compliance program, as an additional element in this process, offers a hospital a further concrete method that may *improve quality of care and reduce waste.* Compliance programs also provide a central coordinating mechanism for furnishing and disseminating information and guidance on applicable federal and state statutes, regulations and other requirements (Section I).

> The OIG recognizes that the health care industry in this country . . . is constantly evolving. However, the time is right for hospitals to implement a strong voluntary compliance program concept in health care. As stated throughout this guidance, *compliance is a dynamic process that helps to ensure that hospitals and other health care providers are better able to fulfill their commitment to ethical behavior,* as well as meet the changes and challenges being imposed upon them by Congress and private insurers (Section III).

This is a more profound view of compliance than that found within the HCCA, one that involves the kinds of moral and social values that could provide a richer notion of professionalism. Of course, if the values themselves are the goal of compliance, rather than just meeting the norms imposed by the OIG, then compliance professionals should question whether the proposed guidelines really meet those values. Do compliance programs, as they are currently conceptualized and practiced, really promote cost-control, elimination of waste, advancement of quality, and the facilitation of ethical behavior? When the costs being externalized to health care institutions are factored in, rather than just focusing on government spending in the short term, are costs really being saved? Do compliance programs, narrowly conceived, eliminate waste and advance quality, or do they divert efforts away from other kinds of efforts toward efficiency and quality that would be more appropriate? Does compliance, with its hotlines and governmental efforts at pitting patient against physician, really advance ethical behavior, or does it rather promote a cynicism about ethics and undermine the very fabric of an ethical culture and life at health care institutions? In all cases, these questions are not even being asked as a part of the compliance movement. There is no research, and no answers are forthcoming. Now compliance must take the next step and directly introduce these concerns. It must shift from a narrow focus on conformity to pre-established norms and directly advance the goals that the OIG associates with compliance; namely, cost-control, elimination of waste, advancement of quality, and the promotion of ethics.

Integration of Compliance and Organizational Ethics

Two facts about the health care context need to be continually kept in mind. First, it is rapidly changing (acknowledged in the OIG Guidelines); second, these changes are such that they call into question long held assumptions about the nature of health care (insufficiently addressed in the OIG guidelines). At the heart of the developments are (1) a web of care (and thus a challenge to the older atomism, with its linear notion of science), (2) an integration of the traditional individual patient orientation with a communal orientation (and thus the challenge of balancing individual and communal interest), and (3) a merging of considerations associated with payment and provision (and thus a move away from a clear disjunct between clinical care and business matters). An organizational ethic is needed to address these changes in a constructive manner. This ethic must be formed at a middle level, between the classical micro-ethic of medical professionalism and the macro-ethic of social policy. Within the compliance movement it is stated that institutions should form their own ethical and business policies, and OIG Guidelines explicitly state that one aspect of compliance should address conformity of practice to institutional ethical guidelines, as well as those of the government. However, in every case, the notion of ethics advanced is one of conformity to pre-established rules. But this misses the character of the organizational ethic that is needed. Just an emphasis on conformity to rules is not needed. Rather, what is needed is the kind of rich ethical reflection that enables current norms to be critically assessed in the light of changing practices, and thus enable these challenges to be worked through. Compliance, conceived as "meeting expectations," can be only one small part of the kind of organizational ethic that is needed.

In practice, however, the tail is continually wagging the dog. Institutions are revisiting mission statements and ethical policies in the light of compliance programs. High priced consultants come in with standardized missions and policies, and these are implemented so that the expectations of external government agents are satisfied. There has not been a rich debate on organizational ethics attending the rapid dissemination of compliance programs.

In the face of this stunted development, there are two options for a more appropriate evolution: (1) a richer notion of compliance, one that moves beyond conformity to rules and incorporates organizational ethics as a constitutive moment of compliance; or (2) compliance, narrowly defined, incorporated as a part of a richer organizational ethic. Either way, an integration of the two must take place. Ethics must become the central focus, and "ethics" must mean more than the narrow, legalistic notion of ethics that is continually found within compliance.

The kinds of considerations that need to be addressed by organizational ethics were outlined earlier in this chapter. The issues to be addressed include the following:

- How are individual and communal interests integrated?
- What is meant by "medically indicated" care, and how is this configured at the institutional level; for example, by guidelines, profiling, etc.?
- How does one equitably address the tradeoffs associated with marginally beneficial care, especially in contexts where there are limited resources available?

- What variability in the standard of care from institution to institution is allowable, especially given the different kinds of missions and values associated with diverse health care institutions?
- Where are norms clear and rational, such that emphasis should be placed upon compliance (for example, clear instances of fraud), and where are they poorly defined and inadequate, such that emphasis should be placed on the formation of alternative norms or policies (for example, areas where rules for billing deviate from the realities of care, are overly cumbersome, or address a rapidly evolving standard of care)?
- What ethical policies best advance quality care, and how does one understand quality?
- Who should be accountable for what areas of practice, and how should the mechanisms of accountability be formulated? (This is especially pressing in areas where teams provide care and there are complex overlapping jurisdictions.)
- How should one understand the new role of administrators in configuring care, and how does one understand institutional agency and accountability? (These two—administrative agency and institutional agency—are linked, but their nature is complex and poorly understood, especially in a context where the majority of legal and ethical norms still assume a neat line between clinical and administrative jurisdictions.)
- How can an institution's legitimate interest in stewardship of resources influence how care is provided? What incentives are appropriate?

These questions are but a small sample of those that need to be asked as a part of an organizational ethic. In nearly every case, compliance documents speak as if these questions have been sufficiently resolved. That, of course, is not the case. Once the values that should direct compliance come to the fore—namely, cost-control, elimination of waste, quality, and ethics—then a body of knowledge needs to be formulated, which is adequate for advancing these values. And that can be done only if these kinds of questions are actively addressed, and if the mechanisms of research and reflection are developed that enable them to be answered.

The Development of a Context Conducive to Open Research and Critical Reflection

To have an organizational ethic, a context is needed that is conducive to the open debate, research, and critical reflection required for the formation of such an ethic. This, perhaps, is one of the greatest challenges facing those in compliance. There is not currently such a context. The question is whether the needed open deliberation is even possible.

When I attended my first HCCA meeting, I was amazed. I had never attended a professional meeting like this before. The closest comparison I can think of is a visit I had to East Berlin before the Iron Curtain came down. In West Berlin there was the kind of vibrancy, lights, noise, and bustle that one finds in any large western city. Then, after passing through the border into East Berlin, there was a thick silence. People would walk with their heads down; everything seemed clean and proper, but there was little life. One could feel the difference in atmosphere. That is what it was like going from all other professional meetings to that compliance meeting. Usually, there is noise, talk, bustle, vibrancy. In this meeting, however, there was a stilted atmosphere. There were no pro and con sessions, no open argument, no critical reflection, no open dissent. This was not in any way a reflection of the efforts of those who organized the conference. The organizers of this event are among the more progressive in the movement—I think the future hope of compliance lies with them. They brought in government representatives to talk, had Federal Bureau of Investigation (FBI) round table discussions, had a plenary session on ethics and an additional breakout session on ethics. To facilitate questioning, they allowed people to submit questions anonymously on cards, so that no one need fear being identified. Despite all of this, however, the atmosphere remained strangely different from other meetings. Two people at that meeting told me that if you ask about a particular code or some other area where you might have a potential compliance violation, then the FBI agents at the meeting write this down, either as a potential area to consider for general investigation, or even as a special area for investigating the institution of the person asking the question. (An FBI agent later told me that this is not true, but that does not change the perception.) One of the leaders in HCCA expressed concern that his or her name was written down by a governmental representative. This was said jokingly, as this person knew it was for a professional reason that the name was written—akin to saying "Wow, you don't want your name before this person"—but it was still indicative of the atmosphere. When at a session I asked a critical question about some of the claims being made on behalf of compliance efforts by the government, three people later came up and told me how they wished that those kinds of issues would be addressed. One of these people was literally whispering his comments to me, and he expressed concern that many people did not feel that they could address their concerns openly. He said that he represents a health care institution, and would fear reprisals to his institution if he openly criticized the way compliance efforts were being advanced. He just wanted to learn how to best address compliance concerns so that his institution does not get in trouble.

Although all compliance meetings may not be like this, even the best of them are not patterned after the model found in other professional organizations. In virtually all cases, compliance meetings are set up as an opportunity to learn what is happening in the cutting edge of compliance (that means: what is being done by the government, and what tools are available for compliance programs). Alternatively, there are introductory sessions that initiate people into the knowledge required. There is no active body of researchers who gather together to exchange information and critically engage the claims that are being made. In fact, no place is even made for such critical analysis. Consultants have a strong interest in seeing a rapid codification of the standards of compliance, and they are often prominently featured in both the leadership of the organization and as speakers at events. Compliance officers at institutions all have a strong professional interest in having their programs recognized as model programs. All of this works against criticism and open debate.

To develop an environment that is conducive to open deliberation, those involved in the organization would need to advance initiatives that work against the immediate economic and prestige interests of the organization. Open deliberation, especially in the controversial areas associated with recent developments in health care, slows things down. A rich discussion on quality would embroil the HCCA in the seemingly interminable debates of outcomes assessment. Discussion of managed care shows how far there is to go before a consensus on the appropriateness of integrating payment and provision is reached. Developing common and statute law shows that we are only in the first stages of holding institutions directly accountable for substandard care, rather than vesting all responsibility for care on the clinicians involved. The current dissent among medical professionals (seen, for example, in the way they view deception of payers as an ethically appropriate option), shows how divergent medical and business ethical models are. It is much easier to assume that those kinds of considerations are external to compliance; that others form the norms that advance quality, cost-control, elimination of waste, and ethics. It is much easier to work with a clear distinction between clinical and business ethics, and import the standards of business ethics and compliance from other sectors of the economy. If those in compliance get involved in the murky areas outlined in this essay, it will undoubtedly derail the rapid development of the field. But it will also lead to a more mature, ethically appropriate notion of compliance.

The choice facing those in compliance is a choice between two fairly clear options. Compliance can be defined narrowly as "meeting the expectations of others," and the body of knowledge can be restricted to those strategies that effectively meet those expectations, especially the ones articulated by government. One can put aside any questions about whether those expectations are appropriate. But then one cannot assume that a clear social or moral value is advanced. This course is undoubtedly preferable, if the interest advanced is one of wealth, influence, and prestige. Alternatively, compliance can be defined in a broader way, advancing the values identified in the OIG Guidelines; namely, the values of cost-control, quality, elimination of waste, and ethics. That, in turn, would require a body of knowledge that assesses whether current standards do actually advance those values. Such knowledge would form slowly, and the process would involve extensive research and controversy. Alliances would need to be formed with other professional organizations, and the power of compliance professionals would be diminished. Then compliance would indeed advance important moral and social values, and one could look to the movement for guidance when addressing the difficult issues that face the nation's health care system.

In the end, the choice is between two forms of professionalism: the narrow, nonmoral one or the moral one. As such, it is a moral choice: between wealth and power, on one side, and the social good, on the other. Anyone making the right choice will have an uphill battle.

NOTES

1. G. Engel, *How Much Longer Must Medicine's View of Science Be Bound By a Seventeenth Century World View?* in THE TASK OF MEDICINE: DIALOGUE AT WICKENBURG 113–36 (K.L. White ed., 1988); G. Engel, *The Need for a New Medical Model: A Challenge for Biomedicine*, 196 SCIENCE 129–36 (1977).

2. The classic account of this scientific foundationalism is found in A. FLEXNER, MEDICAL EDUCATION IN THE UNITED STATES AND CANADA: A REPORT TO THE CARNEGIE FOUNDATION FOR THE ADVANCEMENT OF TEACHING (1910). A detailed assessment of these assumptions is provided in G. Khushf, *Organizational Ethics and the Medical Professional: Reappraising Roles and Responsibilities, in* THE

P<small>HYSICIAN AS</small> F<small>RIEND AND</small> H<small>EALER</small> (J. Kissell & D. Thomasma eds., 2000); and G. Khushf, *What is At Issue in the Debate about Concepts of Health and Disease? Framing the Problem of Demarcation for a Post-Positivist Era of Medicine, in* H<small>EALTH</small>, S<small>CIENCE AND</small> O<small>RDINARY</small> L<small>ANGUAGE</small> 103–51 (L. Nordenfelt ed., 2001).

3. This patient-centered focus can be found throughout the professional ethical literature. Representative essays are M. Angell, *Medicine: The Endangered Patient-Centered Ethic*, 17 H<small>ASTINGS</small> C<small>EN-</small>TER R<small>EP</small>. 12–13 (1987); and E. Pellegrino, *Medical Economics and Medical Ethics: Points of Conflict and Reconciliation*, 69 J. <small>OF</small> MAG 175–83 (Mar. 1980).

4. Much of Flexner's *Medical Education, supra* note 2, involves an attempt to restructure the financing of medical education and practice so that economic considerations are external to practice. The impact of this on the meaning of "medically necessary" care is discussed in G. Khushf, *A Radical Rupture in the Paradigm of Modern Medicine: Conflicts of Interest, Fiduciary Obligations, and the Scientific Ideal*, 23:1 J. M<small>ED</small>. & P<small>HIL</small>. 98–122 (1998).

5. G. Khushf, *Administrative and Organizational Ethics*, 9:4 HEC F<small>ORUM</small> 299–309 (1997).

6. An outstanding discussion of institutions as "silent players" and their recent emergence as active agents can be found in H. M<small>ORREIM</small>, B<small>ALANCING</small> A<small>CT</small>: T<small>HE</small> N<small>EW</small> M<small>EDICAL</small> E<small>THICS OF</small> M<small>EDICINE'S</small> N<small>EW</small> E<small>CONOMICS</small> (1995).

7. H. M<small>ORREIM</small>, B<small>ALANCING</small> A<small>CT</small>: T<small>HE</small> N<small>EW</small> M<small>EDICAL</small> E<small>THICS OF</small> M<small>EDICINE'S</small> N<small>EW</small> E<small>CONOMICS</small> (1995).

8. These and many other recent developments in health care are surveyed in M. R<small>ODWIN</small>, M<small>EDICINE</small>, M<small>ONEY AND</small> M<small>ORALS</small>: P<small>HYSICIAN'S</small> C<small>ONFLICTS OF</small> I<small>NTEREST</small> (1993).

9. D. E<small>DDY</small>, C<small>LINICAL</small> D<small>ECISION</small> M<small>AKING</small>: F<small>ROM</small> T<small>HEORY TO</small> P<small>RACTICE</small>, at 2 (1996).

10. D. E<small>DDY</small>, C<small>LINICAL</small> D<small>ECISION</small> M<small>AKING</small>: F<small>ROM</small> T<small>HEORY TO</small> P<small>RACTICE</small>, ch. 4 (1996).

11. T<small>O</small> E<small>RR IS</small> H<small>UMAN</small>: B<small>UILDING A</small> S<small>AFER</small> H<small>EALTH</small> S<small>YSTEM</small> (L.T. Kohn et al. eds., 2000); for commentary, see T.A. Brennan, *The Institute of Medicine Report on Medical Errors—Could It Do Harm?*, 342:15 N<small>EW</small> E<small>NG</small>. J. M<small>ED</small>. 1123–25 (2000).

12. For a classic review of the impact of technology on medicine, with a concluding chapter on the impact of recent developments on the physician–patient relation, see S.J. R<small>EISER</small>, M<small>EDICINE AND THE</small> R<small>EIGN OF</small> T<small>ECHNOLOGY</small> (1978).

13. H. M<small>ORREIM</small>, B<small>ALANCING</small> A<small>CT</small>: T<small>HE</small> N<small>EW</small> M<small>EDICAL</small> E<small>THICS OF</small> M<small>EDICINE'S</small> N<small>EW</small> E<small>CONOMICS</small> (1995), outlines the two responses and provides an argument in favor of the new role for organizational agents.

14. This approach is well exemplified by E. P<small>ELLEGRINO</small> & D. T<small>HOMASMA</small>, A P<small>HILOSOPHICAL</small> B<small>ASIS OF</small> M<small>EDICAL</small> P<small>RACTICE</small>: T<small>OWARD A</small> P<small>HILOSOPHY AND</small> E<small>THIC OF THE</small> H<small>EALING</small> P<small>ROFESSIONS</small> (1981).

15. This approach is well exemplified in S.M. Shortell et al., *Physicians as Double Agents: Maintaining Trust in an Era of Multiple Accountabilities*, 280:12 JAMA 1102–08 (1998).

16. D.F. Thompson, *Hospital Ethics*, 3 C<small>AMBRIDGE</small> Q. H<small>EALTHCARE</small> E<small>THICS</small> 203–10 (1992); and G. Khushf, *Administrative and Organizational Ethics*, 9:4 HEC F<small>ORUM</small> 299–309 (1997).

17. In a more detailed discussion, the relation between science and complementary and alternative medicine (CAMs) would need to be qualified. These therapies are often responsive to exactly those aspects of illness that are insufficiently addressed within a classical biomedical model, and they involve complex relational factors, which are not easily assessed by traditional scientific methods. Although there may be much that is "unscientific," there are also aspects that may be quite legitimate, but resistant to the way science is currently conceptualized. One thus cannot see CAM as a simple example of unscientific care.

18. G. Engel, *How Much Longer Must Medicine's View of Science Be Bound By a Seventeenth Century World View? in* T<small>HE</small> T<small>ASK OF</small> M<small>EDICINE</small>: D<small>IALOGUE AT</small> W<small>ICKENBURG</small> 113–36 (K.L. White ed., 1988).

19. G. Khushf, *What is At Issue in the Debate about Concepts of Health and Disease? Framing the Problem of Demarcation for a Post-Positivist Era of Medicine, in* HEALTH, SCIENCE AND ORDINARY LANGUAGE 103–51 (L. Nordenfelt ed., 2001).

20. G. Khushf, *A Radical Rupture in the Paradigm of Modern Medicine: Conflicts of Interest, Fiduciary Obligations, and the Scientific Ideal*, 23:1 J. MED. & PHIL. 98–122 (1998).

21. D. KENDIG, PURCHASING POPULATION HEALTH. PAYING FOR THE RESULTS (1997).

22. S.M. Shortell et al., *Physicians as Double Agents: Maintaining Trust in an Era of Multiple Accountabilities*, 280:12 JAMA 1102–08 (1998); *see also* S.H. Miles & R. Koepp, *Comments on the AMA Report: "Ethical Issues in Managed Care,"* 6 J. CLINICAL ETHICS 306–11 (1995).

23. A review of some of these issues is provided in G. Khushf & R. Gifford, *Understanding, Assessing and Managing Conflicts of Interest, in* SURGICAL ETHICS at 342–66 (L. McCullough et al. eds., 1999).

24. The problems of balancing and marginal utility are nicely addressed in D. EDDY, CLINICAL DECISION MAKING: FROM THEORY TO PRACTICE, at 2 (1996). Eddy considers examples from Kaiser's health plans to show how such tradeoffs can be addressed at an organizational level.

25. A good review of these developments is available on the Health Care Financing Administration's Internet site at <http://www.hcfa.gov/medicare/fraud/CMP2.HTM>, and also in the transcript of the National Fraud, Waste and Abuse Conference, March 17, 1998, available on the Internet at <http://www.hcfa.gov/medicare/fraud/transcr7.HTM>.

26. These assumptions are critically assessed in H.T. Engelhardt, *Health Care Reform: A Study in Moral Malfeasance*, 19:5 J. MED. & PHIL. 501–16 (1994); several other essays in this journal issue also attend to the ethical assumptions behind health care reform, especially the need for explicitly addressing the tradeoffs between cost, quality, and access.

27. A common strategy used by both the government and independent compliance consultants proceeds as follows: (1) the size and type of health care institution is determined; (2) using sample data on the percent of claims generally found to be inappropriate, an estimate of the "fraud" at the institution is determined; (3) then a calculation of financial liability to the institution is made, usually resulting in multimillion dollar fines. The institution is told that if it implements a "voluntary" compliance program, this will be taken as a good-faith effort on the part of the institution, and potential fines would be reduced.

28. Consider, for example, the following citation from *Building a Partnership for Effective Compliance: A Report on the Government-Industry Roundtable*, available on the Internet at <http://www.hhs.gov/progorg/oig/modcomp/roundtable.htm>:

> The Government's Assessment of a Compliance Program's Effectiveness. Government participants in the roundtable cited a number of factors to be considered in evaluating the effectiveness of a provider's compliance efforts. Management's commitment to, and good faith efforts to implement, a compliance program may be measured by the funding and legitimate support provided to the function, as well as the background of the individual designated as the compliance officer. Whether there is "buy-in" by the provider's employees and contractors can be influenced by the sufficiency of training and the availability of guidance on policies and procedures. Evidence of open lines of communication and the appropriate use of information lines to address employee concerns and questions was also referenced. A documented practice of refunding of overpayments and self-disclosing incidents of non-compliance with program requirements was also cited as evidence of a meaningful compliance effort by a provider.

29. D.H. Novack et al., *Physicians' Attitudes Toward Using Deception to Resolve Difficult Ethical Problems*, 261:20 JAMA 2980–85 (1989).

30. V.G. Freeman et al., *Lying for Patients: Physician Deception of Third-Party Payers*, 159 ARCHIVES INTERNAL MED. 2263–70 (2000); *see also* D.P. Sulmasy et al., *Physicians' Ethical Beliefs About Cost-Control Arrangements*, 169 ARCHIVES INTERNAL MED. 649–57 (2000).

31. V.G. Freeman et al., *Lying for Patients: Physician Deception of Third-Party Payers*, 159 ARCHIVES INTERNAL MED. 2263 (2000).

32. V.G. Freeman et al., *Lying for Patients: Physician Deception of Third-Party Payers*, 159 ARCHIVES INTERNAL MED. 2269 (2000)

33. V. Foubister, *New Study Confirms: Doctors Willing to Lie for Coverage*, 42 AM. MED. NEWS 1, 29–30 (Nov. 8, 1999).

34. V. Foubister, *New Study Confirms: Doctors Willing to Lie for Coverage*, 42 AM. MED. NEWS 1 (Nov. 8, 1999).

35. Consider, as an example, the following:

    In the context of unprofessional behavior, misrepresentation consists of lying and fraud. . . . [C]onjuring up a diagnosis so that a patient's hospital admission or length of stay can be justified is a lie which insidiously undermines the patient/physician relationship. While the intent may seem to be in the best interest of the patient, the act is not (p. 7).

    AMERICAN BOARD OF INTERNAL MEDICINE, PROJECT PROFESSIONALISM, at 7 (1998).

36. A.S. Brett, *New Guidelines for Coding Physicians' Services—A Step Backward*, 339:23 NEW ENG. J. MED. 1705–08 (1998).

37. A.S. Brett, *New Guidelines for Coding Physicians' Services—A Step Backward*, 339:23 NEW ENG. J. MED. 1706 (1998).

38. A.S. Brett, *New Guidelines for Coding Physicians' Services—A Step Backward*, 339:23 NEW ENG. J. MED. 1708 (1998).

39. A.S. Brett, *New Guidelines for Coding Physicians' Services—A Step Backward*, 339:23 NEW ENG. J. MED. 1707 (1998).

40. For a detailed account of the history of bioethics outlined in this section, *see* A. JONSEN, THE BIRTH OF BIOETHICS (1998).

41. A good overview of the literature associated with ethics committees can be found in THE HEALTHCARE ETHICS COMMITTEE EXPERIENCE: SELECTED READINGS FROM HEC FORUM (S. Spicker ed., 1998).

42. SOCIETY FOR HEALTH AND HUMAN VALUES-SOCIETY FOR BIOETHICS CONSULTATION TASK FORCE ON STANDARDS FOR BIOETHICS CONSULTATION, CORE COMPETENCIES FOR HEALTH CARE ETHICS CONSULTATION (1998).

43. Some of the deficiencies are well addressed in H.T. ENGELHARDT, FOUNDATIONS OF BIOETHICS (2d ed. 1996). Engelhardt notes how bioethicists can function like secular priests, putting forth a bio-ethical orthodoxy as if it represented the considered moral view of all traditions, even when there is significant moral disagreement and ambiguity about the relevant issues. In these cases, bioethics is no better than compliance.

44. In some of the literature on compliance, there is an attempt to focus more broadly on organiza-tional mission and values, rather than just law. This is also highlighted in many OIG documents. However, even in these cases, it is usually assumed that the institution-specific policies and values are like additional laws, and one asks how behavior can conform to this. A rich discussion of virtue and action-guiding ideals is largely absent from the literature.

45. Although few compliance officers are called "Ethics Officers" (the preferred designation is "Cor-porate Compliance Officer"), some still have the language of ethics directly associated with their program or professional title, and nearly all regularly use the language of ethics to advance com-

pliance concerns. In most cases, there is no explicit recognition that there are or should be other programs formally responsible for addressing ethics at the institution, despite the HCCA's explicit statement that "bioethical compliance issues" are separate from the kind of compliance that is addressed by the HCCA.

46. A nice review of the two approaches to professionalism can be found in H.M. Swick, *Toward a Normative Definition of Medical Professionalism*, 75:6 ACADEMIC MED. 612–16 (June 2000).

47. Within the sociological literature, there is an attempt to describe the phenomenon of professionalism without any normative claims regarding its value. Sociologists do not explicitly contrast their approach with those that are morally based; in fact, they often seek to show how even morally oriented accounts of professionalism have a significant element of self-interest. A good example of a sociological analysis of medical professionalism can be found in PAUL STARR'S THE SOCIAL TRANSFORMATION OF AMERICAN MEDICINE (1982). I develop the contrast between the two types of professionalism from a normative ethical perspective, usually with the intent of advocating a form of professionalism that emphasizes ethical ideals. By calling the sociological approach "nonmoral," the aspects of self-interest and power that are identified in those accounts are highlighted.

48. *See* HEALTH CARE COMPLIANCE CERTIFICATION BOARD, CANDIDATE HANDBOOK (2000).

49. A nice review of the government interest in compliance can be found at the American Hospital Association's Web site, in R. Salcido, *The Roles and Responsibilities of Enforcement Agencies*, available on the Internet at <http://www.aha.org/compliance/public-area/rolesresponse.html>.

50. Available on the Internet at <http://www.hcca-info.org>.

51. These sample guidelines can be found in many places; a version is available on the Internet at the American Hospital Association Homepage, <http://www.aha.org/Compliance/Public_Area/toc.html>.

CHAPTER 10

Stress Management for Compliance Professionals

John R. Guetter and Jan C. Heller

INTRODUCTION

This chapter identifies some common sources of work-related stress among compliance professionals as well as some ways to manage that stress productively. It also emphasizes the importance of monitoring departmental and organizational stress, because excessive levels of stress can be associated with some of the problems with which compliance professionals are concerned, including errors, fraud, and sabotage.

For purposes of this discussion, the concept of stress is reserved for those external factors that create discomfort or impair performance. Occupational stress involves factors associated with the job or work conditions that have negative effects on people. The effects of stress on people will be defined as "strain." The psychological and management literatures are very clear in suggesting that under enough stress, people function less effectively—both on and off the job. Empirically, high occupational stress has been linked with higher absenteeism rates, higher error rates, higher accident rates, higher health care costs, lower employee morale, higher employee apathy, increased workplace hostility, increased workplace sabotage, and increased litigation between employees and employers.[1–9]

In fact, the relationship between stress and productivity is generally de-

We are indebted to Samuel Osipow, PhD, and his coworkers who formulated the basic conceptual structure that guided the discussion of occupational stress presented in this chapter. We also thank the many compliance professionals (who shall remain anonymous) for their willingness to share experiences, frustrations, and advice with us.

scribed as "curvilinear."[10] At very low levels of stress, productivity can suffer. Most people appear to need a little stress (that is, external pressure) in order to maintain interest and motivation in their work. However, at higher levels of stress, productivity can also suffer. People then become distracted by their own efforts to cope with stress. In general, moderate levels of stress create an optimal level of arousal that improves motivation and drive without impairing concentration, commitment, or occupational skills.

Decades of research have shown two other important characteristics of stress.[11] First, people vary in their sensitivity to stress. What is stressful for one person might not necessarily be stressful for another. As a result, managers should try to individualize their approaches to employees, providing optimal levels of motivation for each employee. One approach most decidedly does not work for all employees. Second, people vary in their response to stress. One person might become anxious, another might become angry, and yet another person might become physically ill. Despite these differing effects, there is a widely accepted understanding among occupational psychologists that increasing levels of stress from any source produces negative effects, or "strain" in one or more of the following four areas: (1) work performance, (2) psychological functioning, (3) interpersonal relationships, and (4) physical health.

A useful metaphor of the effects of stress involves driving a car. Insufficient external pressure is like driving at 45 miles per hour when the rest of traffic is moving along at 60 miles per hour. When people travel too slowly, they create problems for the rest of traffic that is moving efficiently at 60 miles per hour. They might create a bottleneck, and run the risk of being rear ended by someone who underestimates their speed. Excessive external pressure is like driving 75 miles per hour when the rest of traffic is moving at 60 miles per hour. When people travel too quickly, they may create problems for others who have to dodge or weave to get out of their way. They also have to be very aware of their driving, to monitor any unexpected moves that may require them to slow down quickly. At speeds that are slower or faster than the optimal traffic flow, drivers must be extra aware and careful about the negative impact that their rate of speed may have on themselves or others.

To extend the metaphor a little, occupational stress can also be thought of in terms of the job of an ambulance driver, who must balance competing pressures like traffic and road conditions, patient needs, demands of the emergency medical technicians (EMTs) or paramedics on board, expectations of the driver's boss, and the driver's personal skills, in fulfilling the responsibility to get a patient to a hospital safely and quickly. Ambulance patients, coworkers, and bosses all have some expectations about speed, routes, safety, and manners that drivers must in some way deal with, while the drivers must also maintain responsibility for their vehicles, traffic laws, and public safety. All these demands or expectations influence the drivers' performance, and clearly can increase their levels of stress. In many cases, compliance professionals themselves feel like ambulance drivers. In other cases, they may function more like the ambulance drivers' bosses. In yet other cases, they will be dealing with institutions or organizations in which there are many ambulance drivers and many bosses; their jobs arc to help ensure that all drivers deliver all patients safely and quickly without accidents or traffic violations.

Like traffic conditions for ambulance drivers, work characteristics influence the level of stress experienced by employees. Work that is very precise, demanding, or unusual generally produces a higher level of worker stress than work that is routine, simple, and well practiced. Being asked to transport a patient along a relatively uncrowded highway at 60 miles per hour may be quite appropriate, safe, and not too stressful; being told to do so at the same speed on crowded city streets is hazardous and very stressful! Transporting a critically injured accident victim on crowded city streets is more stressful than transporting a patient with several fractures but who is otherwise stabilized on the same crowded city streets. Compliance professionals should develop a good sense of what is an appropriate speed for the work they have to do; they should have equal sensitivity to the appropriate speeds of the people who work for them, and they should sensitize other health care professionals and managers about appropriate speeds for the work that they do.

EFFECTS OF STRESS

As already noted, stress from any source creates strain for people in at least one of four main ways. Under stress, people may experience vocational strain, psychological strain, interpersonal strain, and physical strain.[12,13]

Vocational strain refers to the effects of stress on actual work performance as well as work-related attitudes and feelings. To apply the driving metaphor, vocational strain happens when external stress impairs ambulance drivers' actual driving skills. They swerve more, brake harder, accelerate more rapidly, and pass more aggressively—all behaviors that increase the possibility of traffic violations or accidents on the way to the hospital.

Usually, health care employees like and are interested in their work, care about their own performance, and feel loyalty to their employers.[14] As they experience higher levels of occupational stress, they might report poorer attitudes toward work, including dread, boredom, and lack of interest. Work quality or quantity may suffer, errors may be made, and difficulties with concentration or attendance may be reported. Higher levels of vocational strain also increase the risk of accidental or deliberate acts of violence, vandalism, carelessness, or illegal and unethical behavior. As a result, vocational strain is one of the effects of stress that can most directly affect compliance professionals and their work in compliance. Unmanaged stress can impair the work of compliance professionals themselves, of their staff, and perhaps most important, of the many employees whose behavior and practices they must monitor or influence.

Psychological strain refers to the effects of stress on people's moods and emotions. In driving terms, ambulance drivers who feel pressured to drive too fast under unsafe conditions may feel or act more anxious, irritable, angry, or impulsive when they are speeding. These emotions may then affect their driving skills, or they may spill over into other parts of their professional or personal lives.

Normally, health care workers report feeling content, flexible, and generally optimistic. They feel satisfied with their lives, are usually free of anxiety, and are good-natured. They do not usually complain about things, and they tend to adapt to problems or interruptions constructively. They usually feel that their lives are "going well." People who are experiencing psychological strain may report feeling anxious, worried, tense, preoccupied, irritable, depressed, or apathetic. They have no sense of humor; may overreact to even small problems; and view themselves as negative, pessimistic, or discouraged. When people experience such negative psychological effects, they are less likely to concentrate, less likely to attend to detail, and more likely to be distracted by their feelings or moods. Although psychological strain does not necessarily lead directly to impaired work performance, clearly it can do so through inattentiveness to detail, more distractibility or preoccupation, and less commitment to work quality.

Interpersonal strain refers to the effects of stress on relationships (for example, with family, close friends, or coworkers). To apply the ambulance metaphor, drivers may become less sociable or friendly with their coworkers, bosses, or even family members when they are expected to drive in ways that they view as unreasonable or unsafe, or if they feel that their driving contributed to a negative effect, such as a patient dying on the way to the hospital.

Under optimal levels of stress, health care workers report no unusual problems with their spouses, family members, friends, or coworkers. They enjoy spending time with others, experience their relationships as generally positive, and usually take a solution-oriented approach to problems in relationships. People who experience high levels of interpersonal strain may report frequent arguments or frustrations in one or more of their close relationships. They may be quarrelsome or excessively sensitive to others. They may want to withdraw and be alone, avoid their friends, or not have many friends. At work, they may be more aloof, more argumentative, less cooperative, or less considerate of the needs and feelings of others.

In health care settings, which tend to be more collegial than hierarchical in communication patterns, interpersonal strain is a concern in at least two ways. First, when managers or directors are stressed, they may express their strain interpersonally toward their coworkers and subordinates. This has a ripple effect, because many people are significantly influenced by their bosses' moods and behavior. Second, when compliance depends, as it often does, on good and clear channels of communication, uncommunicative employees can contribute to problems by their failure to interact and share information that is vital to patient well-being or administrative integrity.

Physical strain refers to the effects of stress on physical health and well-being. This might be like speeding ambulance drivers who get tension headaches or upset stomachs while racing through traffic. Their constant state of high arousal may also contribute to an increased vulnerability to illness or disease.

Normally, health care employees have only occasional concerns about their health; are not often sick; and do not have difficulty with appetite, sleep, or energy levels. People with problems in the physical strain area may report worries about their health as well as physical symptoms or concerns (for example, illnesses, aches and pains, weight changes, sleep problems, overuse of alcohol, feeling lethargic or apathetic). At work, they may have attendance problems, be worried and distracted by their health problems, and generally function less efficiently and effectively.

PERSONAL STRESS MANAGEMENT SKILLS

Improving personal stress management skills generally involves four main skills. First, people should have a way to monitor or assess their level of strain. Second, people should have some ability to identify the stresses that cause them strain. Third, when strain levels are excessive, people should have some ways to reduce or manage the stresses, so that strain is lowered. Finally, if the stresses cannot be modified, people should have some coping skills or techniques that reduce the negative effects of high strain.

Assessing Strain

Good stress management begins with people having a way to assess their personal levels of strain. In driving terms, this is like checking the speedometer and comparing vehicle speed with posted speed limits, surrounding traffic, and road conditions. Although stress assessment is not quite as simple as checking a speedometer, it can be accomplished through one of many ways, including answering questionnaires, using biofeedback or other "psychophysiological" measures, completing stress rating forms, and calculating stress scores.[15–17]

Although there are pros and cons to each approach, a relatively simple approach that psychologists call "scaling" is recommended here. Scaling involves rating on an 11-point scale peoples' subjective sense of their personal strain levels. Essentially, it is suggested that people take a moment to stop *what* they are doing and, instead, think about *how* they are doing. They should take into account how their bodies feel (tense, relaxed, tired, sore, fatigued), how their minds have been working (productively, focused, preoccupied, disorganized, obsessed), what emotional states they have been in (calm, relaxed, tense, irritable, worried, sad, angry, bored), and how they have been acting (rushed, slow, pressured, loud, demanding, touchy). Based on these four dimensions, they rate their overall strain level on a scale of 0 to 10. 0 represents the most calm and relaxed condition they can imagine themselves feeling, and 10 represents the most tense and upset condition they can imagine themselves feeling. The actual strain score usually falls somewhere between those two extremes.

Although it takes some practice to produce reliable ratings, most people find that they can do so within a few days of consistent effort. They become able to distinguish between an overall rating of 4 and 5, or 7 and 8.

Learning to do so provides a way for people to monitor their own strain level, and it helps them to learn what their optimal level of strain actually is. In addition, awareness of their optimal strain level may alert them to times when they should do something to reduce that strain. In practice, most people function most effectively when their strain scores fall somewhere in the 3–5 range. Higher scores lead to increased effort to manage the strain itself, and lower scores may reduce drive and motivation.

Identifying Stress

If people find that their strain levels are too high for their own good, they should then identify the stresses that contribute to their strain. This is like ambulance drivers who know that they are driving too fast (or too slowly) for current road conditions. They may be driving too fast because they feel pressured by their coworkers or by the patients' conditions, because they want to get to their destination to do something important, because they had a fight with a family member, or even because they are preoccupied with personal problems like money, illness, and so forth.

In simplified terms, stress can be divided into personal stress and occupational stress. Personal stress includes any conditions or factors that are associated with people's nonworking lives, including relationship problems, worries about family members, financial or legal concerns, health problems, and a host of other stresses. Although it is beyond the scope of this discussion to review all possible personal stresses, there are several useful resources available to do so.[18–20]

Occupational stress includes those conditions or factors associated with people's working lives, including problems with the work itself or with the conditions (people, policies, procedures) associated with the work. It is helpful to pinpoint the stresses that are contributing to strain, because doing so often helps people to reduce or resolve those stresses. There are several approaches to the analysis of occupational stress. The approach recommended here proposes six factors that are the basic elements of practically any occupation: (1) workload, (2) boredom, (3) role ambiguity, (4) role conflict, (5) responsibility, and (6) work environment.[21,22]

Workload refers to the volume of work people must do. It is influenced by their ability to manage their workloads with their personal and professional skills as well as with their organizational resources and support. Workload stress is like an ambulance driver who is driving faster than the speed limit. It can be dangerous because of the lower margin for error. This is particularly the case if drivers feel pressured to drive at a speed at which they are not comfortable.

One source of workload stress is based on health care workers' skills or abilities. If employees do not know how to do parts of their jobs very efficiently or effectively, tasks will take longer to get done. A second kind of workload stress is based on the sheer amount of work and having too much to do even though employees have adequate skills and abilities. A third kind of overload is caused by workload organization. Some days, weeks, or even months are hectic while others are manageable and perhaps even boringly uneventful. Yet a fourth kind of workload stress is based on work standards—if everything has to be perfect, people will not have nearly as much time to get things done when things only have to be "good enough." A fifth source of workload stress is caused by poor managerial skills. Managers who have difficulty delegating, managers who micromanage the work of others, and managers who "delegate and forget" all may experience workload stress problems.

Health care workers with optimal (that is, ratings in the 3–5 range) stress levels in this area feel that their workloads are reasonable and that they have the skills and resources to do their work. They are reasonably confident that they are competent to complete their assignments and believe that staffing patterns, deadlines, and work schedules are realistic. People with difficulty in this area report that their workloads are increasing, unreasonable, or unsupported by organizational resources. They feel that they are responsible for more work than they can reasonably handle. They may feel inadequately trained or skilled for their jobs. They may believe that the organizational resources are insufficient or inadequate for the work that they must accomplish.

Our formal and informal contacts with compliance professionals suggest that most are responsible for substantial workloads. Although many of them manage their workloads adequately through delegation, personal time management skills, and setting realistic goals, they consistently emphasize that work volume can easily contribute to losing perspective of the "big picture." They credit their previous management experience, support from their own boss or board, and having a good sense of the capabilities of their own staff as key skills in handling their departmental workload.

As managers, successful compliance professionals emphasize the importance of assessing employee workloads frequently, and being sensitive to individual strengths and weaknesses among their employees. As a group, managers tend to underestimate the stress that their employees experience in workload pressure, so they should make allowances for their biased perspective. As a consultant or resource to other departments, the most obvious concern relative to workload is the general tendency for error rates to increase as work volume increases. When employees are confronted with the conflicting pressures of work quantity and work quality, they usually comply with work quantity and take their chances with mistakes not happening or not being caught if they do happen. In some departments, and in some kinds of work, this may be an acceptable compromise; however, in other departments (for example, billing or neurosurgery), this is simply not acceptable. The price for errors is far too high.

Boredom refers to the extent to which people's training, education, skills, and experience match the demands of their work. Boredom stress is like an ambulance driver being required to drive slower than the speed limit even though the roads are clear, visibility is good, traffic is very light, and the patient is stable. One risk of boredom is worker dissatisfaction and demoralization; another is the increased risk for accidents or errors because of carelessness or inattentiveness.

Health care workers with difficulty in this area complain of a sense of boredom, lack of challenge, or underutilization. They may feel that they do not have much of a professional future, or are not adequately recognized for their skills and abilities. For many people, this is quite stressful. In fact, in a study one of us conducted for a private industry, this scale was most highly (negatively) correlated with overall job satisfaction; it was also highly (positively) correlated with vocational strain.[23] Contacts with compliance professionals suggest that although they certainly are not bored, many are also not extremely stimulated by the variety or difficulty of their work. The risk for boredom is higher among members of their staffs, who may be assigned to relatively repetitive, not very challenging duties. It is also higher among members of other departments (for example, billing or pharmacy), where the work becomes quite repetitive and employees feel that they could "do their jobs in their sleep."

Role ambiguity refers to the extent to which people feel that their job priorities, standards, expectations, or evaluation criteria are clear. This kind of stress is like ambulance drivers who do not know what the conditions of their passengers are, which makes it difficult to know how to get to the hospital (for example, whether to take the quickest route, the safest route, or the most reliable route).

Health care employees who have problems in this area are not sure what they are expected to do, how they should be spending their time, or how they will be evaluated. They do not seem to know how to begin on new projects, do not have a clear career plan, and may not know what to do to "get ahead." Contacts with compliance professionals suggest that this is a common source of occupational stress.[24] Health care compliance is a relatively new occupational niche, and expectations about satisfactory professional performance are not always very clear. The most common strategy for coping with role ambiguity has been for compliance professionals to develop their own skills at establishing clarity for themselves, based on their own understanding or interpretation of their host organization's needs, their own skills, and their superiors' expectations.

Role conflict refers to conflict between different superiors, different goals, different priorities, or different expectations. The ambulance drivers who have critically injured patients on board in very congested traffic experience this kind of stress. High density traffic makes drivers tend to slow down to avoid more accidents; critically injured patients make drivers tend to speed up to get them to the hospital more quickly. The conflict between the competing pressures creates stress that can lead to serious performance problems.

Health care workers with problems in this area may have conflicting demands placed on them by different supervisors/managers, or they may feel caught between supervisory demands and organizational goals or priorities, between job demands and personal values or priorities, or between supervisory demands and coworker pressure. They experience conflicting demands and conflicting factions. As a result, they may report that they do not feel proud of what they do, and may not feel much investment in their work or their health care organization. They may also feel unclear about lines of authority and may complain about having more than one person telling them what to do. They may also feel that people are not treated fairly or equally by their managers.

Role conflict is a relatively common source of occupational stress among compliance professionals.[25] They frequently mention being aware of hostility from others about their roles in health care administration. They also struggle with the conflict that arises from the demands of the urgent versus the important. For example, they may have a sense that the most important thing to do is consultation and education with other managers and departments, while the most urgent thing to do is to conduct audits and investigations of identified problems. Compliance professionals also should be sensitive to the conflict people in their own or other departments may have about the compliance functions for which they are responsible. The people who manage this source of stress effectively are quite skilled at reducing their own role ambiguity, addressing role conflict explicitly, garnering organizational support for their sometimes unpopular demands, and most of all, maintaining a realistic perspective that animosity about their roles is usually related to their position, not to themselves as people. Even so, many compliance professionals mentioned the importance of maintaining professional distance between themselves and their organizational peers (with whom they may have conflict) while having access to professional peers in other organizations for support, feedback, and informal consultation about troublesome situations.

Responsibility refers to the stress associated with being responsible for the performance, well-being, and satisfaction of others (for example, subordinates or customers) on the job. This is like the responsibility professional ambulance drivers have for the safety and satisfaction of their passengers (both the injured ones and the EMTs or paramedics on board). Failure may result in complaints and perhaps even accidents or deaths.

Health care employees usually believe that the level of responsibility they have is reasonable for their positions. People who report high stress in this area feel frustrated with a sense responsibility for things or people over whom they have little control or influence. They report excessively high levels of responsibility for the work of others, may be worried that others will not perform well, and may be sought out for leadership or assistance that they feel unqualified or unable to provide. They may complain of poor relationships with people at work, or may feel that they have to work with difficult people.

Our experience and contacts indicate that most compliance professionals have a staff that they must manage; many also work with employees over whom they have no direct administrative authority. Rarely is this aspect of managerial responsibility identified as a significant source of stress. However, most compliance professionals do acknowledge that their indirect responsibility for the appropriate conduct of a large number of health care providers and employees that they do not even know can be stressful. Typically, successful compliance professionals cope with this by concentrating on what they can control (for example, developing monitoring systems that work, gaining input from people at all levels of the organization, or collaborating with others to develop positive incentives for compliance) while deemphasizing what they cannot control.

Work environment refers to stresses associated with physical conditions such as excessive noise, pollutants, or heat. This is like driving an ambulance with poor brakes and no air conditioning on a hot day through the crowded streets. Work environment also refers to the social and political factors associated with the organizations in which people work. These social and political factors are sometimes discussed as organizational climate and culture.[26] *Organizational climate* refers to the feeling that is communicated by an organization's physical layout and by the way members of the organization typically interact with each other and with outsiders.[27] *Organizational culture* is the more comprehensive of the two terms (that is, a consideration of culture includes climate), and at its most basic level it refers to the accumulated shared learnings or assumptions that an organization builds up over time as it solves internal and external problems related to its existence.[28] Organizational culture tells members not only how they should feel (as climate does), but also the correct way to perceive and to think in relation to those problems of existence. These shared learnings or assumptions are taught to new members, symbolized in rituals and stories, and are exemplified in important leaders, especially the founders of the organization.

The relationship between organizational climate and culture and the behaviors associated with a stressful work environment is indirect, but culture can certainly influence behavior.[29-31] In terms of the ambulance analogy, it would be like working for an ambulance company in which the informal expectation among drivers is to provide speedy service even if safety is risked. The bravado of risk-taking and close calls may influence an otherwise responsible driver to take unreasonable chances on the job. There are assumptions built into organizational cultures that influence the level of stress that is experienced by employees. The ability to work in or "handle" high-stress cultures may even be an explicit expectation, as in some start-up "dot.com" companies.

Health care workers with problems in this area complain of exposure to hazardous or stressful work conditions, and they may be worried about the effects of these factors on their health or well-being. They may complain of erratic work schedules or of feeling personally isolated. They may complain about unfair treatment, favoritism or discriminatory practices, emotional abuse, or workplace bullying. They may also feel pressure to ignore illegal or unethical practices by their peers or managers. Although most compliance professionals were not very concerned about the physical aspects of their work environments, they consistently identified stress associated with the organizational cultures (the social and political environments) in which they worked. Because much of what compliance professionals do is to influence how other people do their work, they consistently rate the ability to figure out ways to get things done through other people as one of their most important stress management skills.

As mentioned, previous contacts with compliance professionals have suggested that the primary sources of occupational stress for them have been role ambiguity, role conflict, and work environment.[32] As a relatively new professional role within health care settings, compliance professionals often struggle with the fact that their role is not very clear, even to themselves. Although they may have colleagues in similar settings, the role expectations and institutional priorities are not necessarily the same; therefore, doing what their colleagues do is not necessarily an appropriate way to reduce ambiguity. Recent surveys of compliance professionals suggest that they must perform at least three overlapping functions: a consulting/educational function to increase awareness of "doing things right," an investigative function to ensure compliance and censure wrongdoing, and a risk management function to develop strategies and systems to minimize exposure and maximize the likelihood that things will be done right.[33] It may be helpful to prioritize these emphases in individual settings to help manage the ambiguity of the compliance role.

Role conflict is potentially the most serious source of professional stress for compliance professionals. The conflict is often between their own expectations and the expectations of people in other departments. In health care settings, which tend to be administratively decentralized, compliance professionals are likely to find themselves coping with multiple conflicting expectations, which may vary from high levels of congruence and cooperation on one extreme to high levels of resistance and resentment on the other. Shifting among multiple groups with diverse expectations and attitudes can itself be quite stressful.

The social and political environment is the third area that has been consistently stressful for compliance professionals. Like many senior-level positions, compliance involves getting things done through people and departments over which the compliance professional has no direct control. Further, these tasks must get done despite competing pressures from peers whose priorities are frequently different than those of compliance professionals. This requires a high level of interpersonal skill, as it is almost always easier to accomplish goals if compliance professionals can get people to cooperate voluntarily. It requires "cultural skills" in remaining flexible and respectful about how things get done while ensuring that what gets done complies with relevant regulations and laws. It also requires the political skills to identify who the "opinion leaders" are whose cooperation counts most, and in some cases, to know when they should "pull rank" by getting support from their bosses or boards in order to insist on cooperation from people who are genuinely opposed to the compliance professionals' basic goals and priorities.

Alternatives for Personal Stress Reduction

The third step in occupational stress management is stress reduction. In general terms, there are three basic approaches to reduce the negative effects of stress. When possible, the easiest approach is to reduce the stress itself. When that is not possible or not enough, a second approach is to devise strategies that offset the negative effects of stress. When even that is not possible or not enough, the third, and often most difficult, approach is to develop ways to become more "stress-hardy;" that is, to reduce people's sensitivity to stress.

The first approach is to reduce stress. As discussed earlier, *workload* refers to the amount of work for which people are responsible. People for whom this is a primary source of stress often benefit from clarifying what a reasonable workload is, planning ahead to anticipate changing workloads, negotiating with their managers about hiring extra help, learning to delegate more appropriately, establishing more realistic performance standards for themselves, receiving additional training in time management skills or in technical or professional skills, or in some cases, arranging for a reduction in their responsibilities.[34,35]

Boredom refers to the level of interest, challenge, and complexity of people's work. People for whom this is a primary source of stress often benefit from job enrichment, job expansion, or job promotion. These options are frequently worth exploring with their managers. If these are not realistic options, people might explore another career or employer. If these are also not realistic options, then they might explore compensating for their occupational boredom by pursuing hobbies, community service, or other activities away from work that may increase a personal sense of fulfillment. If people cannot change their jobs, they might try a different attitude or perspective. When they focus on what the job does provide (for example, income, stability, security, and freedom to pursue outside interests), it may help them cope with their boredom.

Role ambiguity refers to the extent to which peoples' job expectations are clear and consistent. People for whom this is a primary source of stress often benefit from developing or reviewing their job description, getting clarification from their managers about what they expect, working with an internal or an external mentor or coach to help them clarify job priorities, or proposing clear goals themselves. If ambiguity is part of the job, it can be helpful for people to remind themselves of that, and to check with others about how they cope with ambiguity.

Role conflict refers to conflict between different superiors, goals, priorities, or expectations. People with difficulty in this area often benefit from working with their managers to resolve role conflicts or setting priorities when decisions must be made. If there are contradictory responsibilities among multiple supervisors, people sometimes benefit by asking them to come together to develop ways to resolve those contradictions or to prioritize what should be done when there is a conflict. If the conflict is between what people expect of themselves and what their supervisors expect of them, they should discuss this with their supervisors, if possible. If this is not possible (for example, if the supervisor is part of the problem), they should consider getting input or support from a mentor, a career coach, or a professional colleague.

Responsibility refers to the stress associated with the performance, well-being, and satisfaction of others on the job. People with difficulty in this area often benefit from training in leadership, management, or supervisory skills; from consulting with their own or other managers about ways of handling people; from coaching by a peer or a consultant; or from reviewing their own management style to ensure that they plan, organize, delegate, and follow-up with people in ways their work group needs. In some cases, they can benefit from recognizing that they assume too much responsibility for problems or projects that they cannot control.

Work environment refers to stresses associated with physical, social, and political factors in the workplace. People who have problems in this area often benefit from taking physical precautions to ensure safety, working with managers to make appropriate environmental modifications, or working with their human resource departments to correct grossly inappropriate or unfair employment practices. People who are relatively inexperienced in the social and political aspects of executive work frequently benefit from having internal or external mentors who can help them understand how things get done in their organizations. Environmental conditions that cannot be changed require employees to adjust their expectations or attitudes to cope with those conditions. A consistent finding in the organizational literature is that worker perceptions of their work environment are strongly influenced by the experience they have with their own supervisors or managers.[36] Thus, managers should try hard to ensure that the work environment of their employees is fair, reasonable, and positive.

The second approach is to develop alternative coping resources. It is usually simplest to correct or resolve the workplace stresses that cause strain on employees; however, it is not always possible to do so. Some positions are inherently ambiguous, conflicted, or boring. Other positions may not be inherently stressful, but the organizational ability or will to reduce the stresses may not exist. If the stress cannot be reduced, employees can consider the alternative of using coping techniques that offset the negative effects of occupational stress. In general terms, there are four main groups of coping techniques that many people find helpful: (1) recreation, (2) self-care, (3) social support, and (4) cognitive coping skills.[37,38]

Recreation refers to a willingness and ability to do things that people find relaxing and enjoyable. The key issue is to find activities that people genuinely enjoy, not ones that others would necessarily enjoy. Normally, people report that they take advantage of opportunities to pursue personal interests and relaxing activities. They feel that they can maintain a sensible balance between work demands and personal time. People with problems in this area report not having many interests or not taking the time for the interests they do have. They do not have activities that provide recreation, relaxation, and stress-reduction for themselves. They often benefit by using one or more of the following strategies: They might take a few days off or plan an active but relaxing vacation with some distracting activities to take their minds off work. They might commit some time to do things they really enjoy. They might list the things they most enjoy doing, then pick one or two, and make a point of doing them soon. They might join a club, team, or group with a regular schedule of activities that they enjoy. They might set aside time during the week, when they are not at work, that is scheduled specifically for some sort of recreational activity. For those who have difficulty identifying recreational interests, they might take a survey to identify activities or interests that they might enjoy.

Self-care refers to personal habits that are healthy and that help reduce the effects of chronic or ongoing stress. These include activities such as getting regular exercise, getting enough restful sleep, eating sensibly, relaxing, and avoiding harmful substances (excess alcohol, tobacco, caffeine, or other drugs). People with problems in this area report not getting enough exercise, rest, or relaxation, and may acknowledge using alcohol, cigarettes, coffee, or other drugs excessively. They often benefit from one or more of the following strategies: They might set aside some time to complete a careful review of their personal habits. They might ask a family member or close friend to offer an objective opinion of their self-care habits. They might schedule a physical exam and discuss with their physician some strategies for improving their health. They might try to limit their consumption of caffeinated beverages, alcohol, cigarettes, and nonprescription drugs. They might review their sleep pattern to ensure that they are getting enough sleep. They might modify their diets by reducing portion size or their tendency to snack. They might start to exercise consistently. (An exercise plan should have as high a priority as work. They should plan exercise programs that they can maintain and that are appropriate for their physical conditions.) They might also try relaxation techniques such as meditation, deep breathing, body massage, soaking in spas or warm baths, or muscle relaxation.

Social support refers to the extent to which people feel support and help from people around them. Normally, people feel that there are others who care about them, who would support them if they needed it, who are sympathetic to their problems, and with whom they can talk about solutions to work and life problems. People with problems in this area are alienated, feel even their friends do not care or understand them, or they might be isolated individuals with no friends to talk with or turn to. They often benefit from one or more of the following strategies: They might talk to people (family, friends, or peers) they care about and who care about them and share specifics about their work or other stressful situations. They might try to establish a closer relationship with their bosses. (Research has shown that a positive relationship with one's supervisors can be the most important source of support in the work environment.[39]) If people have become isolated, they might try to expand their network of friends by joining groups, clubs, or organizations that sponsor activities in which they have an interest.

Cognitive coping refers to the logical, systematic techniques people can use to solve professional or personal problems. Normally, people use problem-solving techniques such as defining the problem, considering alternatives, anticipating consequences for self and others, and setting priorities before they take action. They are able to avoid distraction, they can adapt to new information or demands, and they can put the job out of their minds when they go home. They tend to be positive, optimistic, and believe that they can handle most of they problems they face. People with problems in this area have difficulty dealing with unexpected problems, and tend to use techniques to avoid facing or dealing with problems. They may panic or become angry or explosive. They may also ignore problems until someone else has to deal with them. They may solve problems impulsively, and create more problems for themselves by doing so. They have difficulty setting priorities, and are inflexible in adapting to new information or new conditions. People with problems in this area often benefit from following the discipline of a work schedule, evaluating new assignments in relation to existing priorities, giving themselves permission to say "no," to delegate, consulting with a peer or boss, or thinking about a problem before taking action to fix it. They may also benefit from reading books or taking workshops in time management, conflict management, positive or optimistic thinking, or problem-solving skills.[40-43]

Our informal contacts and experience with compliance professionals have consistently endorsed all of these coping strategies as helpful. In particular, compliance professionals report the importance of social support to counteract the tendency to be somewhat isolated organizationally. Senior executive positions tend to be ones in which there is a high level of interaction without very much explicit support. The institutional assumption often is that people at senior levels should not need things like support from their colleagues. In addition, senior executives often work in a fairly competitive environment in which too much sharing might be viewed as a weakness. Regardless, most compliance professionals have emphasized the importance of having one or a few people who care, who are willing to listen, and in some cases, who might be willing to help think about ways to deal with complex situations.

In addition, executives in general, and compliance professionals in particular, have jobs that demand a high level of mental activity without much physical activity. Compliance professionals get paid to think! As a result, they frequently find that a structured routine of vigorous physical activity is essential in maintaining a sense of well-being and balance, and to combat the sedentary aspects of their professional life.

A third general stress management approach is to increase stress tolerance, which has the effect of reducing people's experience of strain.[44] As suggested earlier, people vary in their sensitivity to stress, and in some cases it is not practical or possible to reduce or offset stress. However, in situations when this approach is desirable, there are ways to become more "stress-hardy"; that is, to reduce people's sensitivity to stress, by reducing vocational, psychological, interpersonal, or physical strain, even if the stresses remain the same.

To review briefly, *vocational strain* refers to the negative effects of stress (from any source) on actual work performance as well as work-related attitudes and feelings. When stress negatively affects work, underlying problems with work may be part of the reason. People who wish to reduce vocational strain may benefit by discussing their personal career plans and goals with their boss, a mentor, or a career coach. Such discussion may help put their current strain in a larger and more manageable perspective. Out of this may come an increased commitment to their current jobs. What might also happen is some negotiation about a change in responsibilities, or perhaps even a career change. If the vocational strain is a result of personal stress, consultation with a counselor or mental health professional might be appropriate in pinpointing the sources of stress and developing a plan to reduce it. From a compliance perspective, it is important to be aware of the risks associated with unrecognized vocational strain, and to encourage constructive ways for managers to recognize and address it among their employees. As managers, it is equally important for compliance professionals to "have their own houses in order" by monitoring and addressing vocational strain in their own staff. When vocational strain is a departmentwide problem, managers might consider strategies such as team-building (to increase productive communication and problem-solving), consultation (to identify other sources of departmental stress, including perhaps their own leadership style), or morale-boosting activities (to increase employees experience of work being fun as well as serious).[45-49]

Psychological strain refers to the negative effects of stress on people's emotions and moods. Increasing levels of stress (from any source) makes some people more anxious, depressed, or irritable. People who wish to reduce their own psychological strain might benefit from reading a self-help book about anxiety, depression, or anger.[50,51] They might also benefit from cultivating a sense of humor by exposure to comedy through books, movies, jokes, television shows, and so on. Often people who experience psychological strain benefit from talking with a supportive friend—just "talking about it" seems to help many people. In some cases, medicines to reduce anxiety or depressed moods can be very helpful; in other cases, counseling or psychotherapy can be just as effective. Consultation with a physician or mental health professional can be helpful in clarifying these treatment alternatives.

From a managerial perspective, psychological strain has a tendency to impair performance, and when unaddressed, anxious or depressed individuals can be demoralizing to their coworkers. Managers should be aware of resources available to help them as well as their employees in such cases, including consultation with human resource and employee assistance professionals, as well as with experienced and wise peers.

Interpersonal strain refers to the extent to which people respond to external stress by changing their styles of relating to people close to them, including family members, friends, or coworkers. People may respond to stress by resorting to two main interpersonal patterns: (1) withdrawing from significant relationships and isolating themselves, and (2) taking out their frustrations on people close to them—they become more aggressive and can become a source of stress themselves! People who wish to reduce their level of interpersonal strain might benefit from a conscious examination of their relationships. People who tend to withdraw might schedule time with family or friends even if they do not feel like doing so. They might try to push themselves to talk and share their thoughts and feelings with a supportive family member or friend. If they cannot share their concerns, they might at least spend time doing mutually enjoyable activities. People who become aggressive under stress might try to set firm limits on their own tendency to yell, to criticize, or to become demanding. They might try to keep score on themselves, counting the number of times when they restrained the urge to act aggressively. Better yet, they might share their goal with a spouse, partner, or close friend who will support their efforts to be more considerate, even when things are stressful.

Physical strain refers to people's health problems and their health habits. In response to stress, some people actually become more symptomatic (experiencing colds, heart palpitations, aches and pains, sleep disturbances, or fatigue) and vulnerable to stress-related illnesses.[52–54] Other people tend to neglect their health habits such as sensible diet, regular exercise, adequate sleep, and time to relax. They may also abuse alcohol or other drugs. People who wish to reduce their physical strain might benefit from one or more of the following strategies. They might consult their personal physician to complete a thorough physical examination. They should review appropriate plans for diet and exercise. If they tend to eat too much of the wrong foods, they might develop a plan to cut down on foods with too much salt, sugar, or fat. If they drink too much or smoke too much, they might develop a plan to cut down or stop altogether. If sleep is a problem, they should make sure they schedule enough time to sleep, based on their own sleep needs. Exercise programs may help improve sleep as well as contribute to overall physical health.

MANAGING DEPARTMENTAL STRESS

Compliance professionals usually have people working for them in their departments. They may also have personnel loaned to them from other departments for specific projects. As managers, it is important for them to manage not only their own stress, but to be aware of and manage the occupational stress of the people who work for them. The discussion so far has suggested that one stress management strategy involves working with one's boss.

When compliance professionals are the bosses, however, they should be prepared to respond to the stress-related problems of their employees. Even better, they should try to create a departmental climate that fosters an optimal level of stress for their staff; they can thereby provide a model of how other departments can work more effectively. As leaders in their own departments, they can also influence the culture of their departments. Recall that organizational culture refers to shared learnings or assumptions that an organization develops as it solves internal and external problems related to its existence. These organizational learnings may be largely shared on the departmental level or departmental cultures may be different in varying degrees—this will vary from organization to organization and from department to department. In any case, if leaders want to influence their own stress and that of their employees, they will need to understand their organizational and departmental cultures in order to use their cultures to solve problems for their employees. For instance, regardless of what policies permit, does the culture allow employees to take family leave when a child or spouse is sick? Does the culture tolerate work left undone at the end of the 40-hour workweek when generally productive employees have already worked more than 45 hours? Most important for compliance professionals, does the culture make it easy to do the right thing when a problem is uncovered, or does it "shoot the messenger" (that is, the compliance staff)? How managers structure their own department's climate and culture can model to others a better way to work.

Assessing Departmental Stress

As managers, compliance professionals should be aware of the working conditions of the people they manage. This, of course, includes the occupational stresses experienced by these people. There are several ways of doing this. Probably the most common, and most important, is to be in regular contact with employees, so that they can tell their managers about their needs or concerns. MBWA ("management by walking around") is still a good way to get a sense of the day-to-day atmosphere of a department, particularly if managers are sensitive to issues like optimal working conditions.

Unfortunately, managers consistently underestimate how stressful they and their departments are to work for, and this is the problem with managers using their own impressions of the stresses in their departments. As a generalization, managers almost uniformly believe they are more accessible, more fair, and more aware of worker concerns than their subordinates believe. Managers also tend to underestimate the impact of their own role as boss in influencing how they view themselves and their employees. There are several ways to correct for this bias. First, it is very helpful to ask employees about their perceptions. Employees often do not volunteer information that they believe their bosses might not like unless they are asked explicitly. Second, the information managers get is more likely to be valid if people are assured that there will be no adverse consequences for what they disclose. Third, providing anonymity in completing questionnaires or surveys increases the likelihood of getting such information. Fourth, initiating a team-building process for the purpose of improved work conditions for the entire work group can help create honest input. Most important, however, workers observe how their managers respond to input that they already receive. No matter how often managers say that they want input and honest communication, if they fail to use the input they already received, then their employees will tend not to provide more.

Based on their assessment of work-related stress, compliance professionals may find one of three main conditions in their departments. First, they may find that there are no stress-related problems. Second, they may find that there are some problems, but that the problems are isolated and related to individual workers and their ways of handling stress. Third, they may find that there are departmentwide problems that most or all employees identify as sources of stress. Compliance professionals who have no individual or departmental problems may have found some managerial secrets that would be worth sharing with other compliance professionals or other department heads! These cases are rare, but they do happen.

Managing Departmental Stress

In most cases, compliance professionals will find that there are at least some individuals who have problems with stressful working conditions. In these cases, their first responsibility as managers is to understand the individuals in their departments well enough to know how to help them work at optimal levels. Sometimes, managers assume that their employees have more job training or skills than they actually have. Other times, managers underestimate their employees' need for structure, support, or even encouragement from their bosses. The trickiest situations occur when managers underestimate the (negative) impact they have on their own employees. Based on their understanding of the individuals and their needs, managers should then evaluate what they can do in terms of structure, support, policies, expectations, or managerial style to assist their highly stressed employees to feel less stressed and become more productive.

Sometimes, compliance professionals will find that their entire departments are stressed and functioning poorly. In these situations, they should try to identify common themes that most or all employees identify as stressful. Employees themselves often have a pretty good idea about what creates stress for them, and so managers can use individual or group techniques to identify and prioritize those stresses. Another alternative is to administer questionnaires that identify occupational stresses, and combine individual results into group profiles. One or more of the occupational stresses previously outlined is likely to emerge, and managers can then use some of the guidelines already presented to modify their departmental work environment. They could include policy changes, personnel changes, training, or morale-boosting activities.

MANAGING ORGANIZATIONAL STRESS

When compliance professionals are sensitive to the potentially negative effects of individual and departmental stress, they also become more attuned to stress levels in other departments. Occasionally, they might be working in a health care setting in which the entire organization is experiencing stress. More often, they will find that one or more departments within the overall organization are experiencing higher levels of stress, which increase the risk for errors, mistakes, and problems in those departments. Organizationwide problems are most likely to occur when there are pervasive environmental problems such as changes in health care financing mechanisms (such as the change from indemnity insurers to health maintenance organizations) or significant changes in institutional identity (such as being bought or sold by another organization). Organizationwide stress also can occur when there are serious problems with organizational leadership, fiscal soundness, or organizational culture. In these cases, compliance professionals may not be the people who make the changes, but they may be instrumental in identifying the risks associated with organizationwide stress.[55,56] They may then help the organization's leadership team (of which they are a part) to identify and remedy the stresses. When there is an organizationwide tendency to create stressful working conditions such as workload, role ambiguity, or responsibility, the organization's leaders might consider implementing some of the strategies reviewed earlier.

CONCLUSION

Compliance professionals are responsible for helping to ensure the integrity of the organizations that employ them. Many factors influence that integrity, and many of them are considered in other chapters in this book. This chapter makes the case that personal and occupational stress influence work integrity at all levels of all organizations. Compliance professionals have a responsibility to be sensitive to the negative effects of stress throughout their organizations. They should certainly be sensitive to the effects of stress on their own jobs, as they can be quite stressful. They should be sensitive to the effects of stress on the employees in their own departments. They should also be sensitive to, and sensitize other managers to, the effects of stress in other departments.

Beyond making the case that stress matters, this chapter has provided a conceptual framework for understanding occupational stress. Pinpointing sources of stress such as workload, boredom, ambiguity, role conflict, responsibility, and environmental stress can help people devise ways to manage those stresses. Once the sources of stress are clarified, be they for individuals, departments, or entire organizations, this chapter presented three main strategies for managing occupational stress. First, specific stresses can sometimes be titrated up or down, depending on the needs of the individuals or departments. Second, if the stresses cannot be modified, individuals or departments can be encouraged to develop coping skills to offset the negative effects of stress, including the use of recreation, self-care, social support, and rational coping skills. Third, individuals or departments can be helped to become more skilled in tolerating stress, by reducing their vulnerability to vocational, psychological, social, or physical strain.

NOTES

1. C. Cooper & J. Marshall, *Occupational Sources of Stress: A Review of the Literature Relating to Coronary Heart Disease and Mental Ill Health*, 49:1 J. OCCUPATIONAL PSYCHOL. 11–28 (1976).

2. J. Hurell & L. Murphy, *An Overview of Occupational Stress and Health, in* ENVIRONMENTAL AND OCCUPATIONAL MEDICINE, SECOND EDITION 675–84 (W.M. Rom ed., 1992).

3. F. Landy et al., *Work Stress and Well Being*, 1:1 INT'L J. STRESS MGMT. 33–73 (1994).

4. D.C. Ganster & J. Schaubroeck, *Work Stress and Employee Health*, 17:4 J. OF MGMT. 235–71 (1991).

5. J.M. IVANCEVICH & M.T. MATTESON, STRESS AND WORK: A MANAGERIAL PERSPECTIVE (1980).

6. M.R. Manning et al., *Occupational Stress and Health Care Use*, 1:1 J. OCCUPATIONAL HEALTH PSYCHOL. 100–09 (1996).

7. L. Levi, *Occupational Stress: Spice of Life or Kiss of Death?*, 45:10 AM. PSYCHOLOGIST 1142–45 (1990).

8. T.A. Beehr & J.E. Newman, *Job Stress, Employee Health and Organizational Effectiveness: A Facet Analysis, Model and Literature Review*, 31:6 PERSONNEL PSYCHOL. 665–99 (1978).

9. C. Ostroff, *The Relationship Between Satisfaction, Attitudes, and Performance: An Organizational Level Analysis*, 77:6 J. APPLIED PSYCHOL. 963–74 (1992).

10. A.J. SANFORD, COGNITION AND COGNITIVE PSYCHOLOGY (1985).

11. R.B. Kolbell, *When Relaxation Is Not Enough, in* JOB STRESS INTERVENTIONS 31–43 (L.R. Murphy et al. eds., 1995).

12. S.A. Osipow et al., *Occupational Stress, Strain, and Coping Across the Life-span*, 32:1 J. VOCATIONAL BEHAVIOR 1–15 (1985).

13. S.H. OSIPOW, OCCUPATIONAL STRESS INVENTORY REVISED EDITION (OSI-R) PROFESSIONAL MANUAL (1998).

14. In this and the sections that follow, we describe characteristics of high, normal, and excessive levels of strain and stress among health care workers. These characterizations are extrapolations based on observations and empirical work done with employees in various industries, especially by S.H. Osipow and A.S. Davis, *The Relationship of Coping Resources to Occupational Stress and Strain*, 32:1 J. VOCATIONAL BEHAVIOR 1–15 (1988), S.H. Osipow and A.R. Spokane, *Measuring Occupational Stress, Strain, and Coping*, in APPLIED SOCIAL PSYCHOLOGY ANNUAL REVIEW 5 67–87 (1984) (S. Oskamp ed., 19), C. Ostroff, *The Relationship Between Satisfaction, Attitudes, and Performance: An Organizational Level Analysis*, 77:3 J. APPLIED PSYCHOL. 963–74 (1992), and J.J. Hurrell et al., *Measuring Job Stressors and Strains: Where We Have Been, Where We Are, and Where We Need To Go*, 3:4 J. OCCUPATIONAL HEALTH PSYCHOL. 368–89 (1998), among others. There has been a dearth of empirical work specifically assessing health care workers using the approach we discuss in this chapter, and in fact, we view this as a knowledge gap that should be filled. Absent such specific empirical work however, we believe, based on our own experiences with health care workers and health care systems, that the characterizations we provide are reasonably accurate descriptions of the work conditions within the health care industry.

15. R.S. LAZARUS & S. FOLKMAN, STRESS APPRAISAL AND COPING (1984).

16. H. Hinds & W. Burroughs, *How to Know When You're Stressed: Self-Evaluations of Stress*, 124:1 J. GEN. PSYCHOL. 105–11 (1997).

17. J.J. Hurrell et al., *Measuring Job Stressors and Strains: Where We Have Been, Where We Are, and Where We Need to Go*, 3:4 J. OCCUPATIONAL HEALTH PSYCHOL. 368–89 (1998).

18. R.H. MOOS, LIFE STRESSORS AND SOCIAL RESOURCES INVENTORY PROFESSIONAL MANUAL (1994).

19. R.S. LAZARUS & S. FOLKMAN, STRESS APPRAISAL AND COPING (1984).

20. W.D. ANTON & J.R. REED, EAPI: EMPLOYEE ASSISTANCE PROGRAM INVENTORY PROFESSIONAL MANUAL (1994).

21. S.H. OSIPOW & A.R. SPOKANE, OCCUPATIONAL STRESS INVENTORY MANUAL RESEARCH VERSION 1–5 (1992).

22. S.H. OSIPOW, OCCUPATIONAL STRESS INVENTORY 12 (rev. ed. 1998).

23. J.R. Guetter, OSI-R Data for EAPI and CASI Concurrent Validity Study (1997) (unpublished raw data; contact author for more information).

24. J.C. Heller & J.R. Guetter, *Is Compliance Officer a Tough Job or What?* 1:3 J. HEALTH CARE COMPLIANCE 45–50 (1999).

25. Heller & Guetter (1999).

26. M. Peterson, *Work, Corporate Culture, and Stress: Implications for Worksite Health Promotion*, 21:4 AM. J. HEALTH BEHAVIOR 243–52 (1997).

27. E.H. SCHEIN, ORGANIZATIONAL CULTURE AND LEADERSHIP 9 (2d ed. 1992).

28. E.H. SCHEIN, ORGANIZATIONAL CULTURE AND LEADERSHIP 10 (2d ed. 1992).

29. S. Cartwright et al., *Diagnosing a Healthy Organization: A Proactive Approach to Stress in the Workplace*, in JOB STRESS INTERVENTIONS 217–34 (L.R. Murphy et al. eds., 1995).

30. M. Peterson, *Work, Corporate Culture, and Stress: Implications for Worksite Health Promotion*, 21:4 AM. J. HEALTH BEHAVIOR 243–52 (1997).

31. C. Ostroff, *The Relationship Between Satisfaction, Attitudes, and Performance: An Organizational Level Analysis*, 77:6 J. APPLIED PSYCHOL. 963–74 (1992).

32. Heller & Guetter (1999).

33. See Chapter 3, *A Model for the Compliance Professional: Consulting, Policing, and Managing.*

34. S. Schurman & B. Israel, *Redesigning Work Systems to Reduce Stress: A Participatory Action Research Approach to Creating Change, in* JOB STRESS INTERVENTIONS 235–63 (L.R. Murphy et al. eds., 1995).

35. P. Moyle, *Longitudinal Influences of Managerial Support on Employee Well-Being*, 12:1 WORK & STRESS 29–49 (1998).

36. S.H. Osipow & A.S. Davis, *The Relationship of Coping Resources to Occupational Stress and Strain*, 30 JOURNAL OF EMPLOYMENT COUNSELING 79–87. See also M. CUNNINGHAM & C. COFFMAN, FIRST, BREAK ALL THE RULES (1999), D. Ganster, *Interventions for Building Healthy Organizations: Suggestions from the Stress Research Literature, in* JOB STRESS INTERVENTIONS 323–336 (L.R. Murphy et al. eds., 1995), P. Moyle, *Longitudinal Influences of Managerial Support on Employee Well-Being*, 12:1 WORK & STRESS 29–49 (1998) and S.L Kirmeyer & T.W. Dougherty, *Work Load, Tension, and Coping: Moderating Effects of Supervisor Support*, 41:2 PERSONNEL PSYCHOL. 125–39 (1988).

37. S.H. Osipow & A.S. Davis, *The Relationship of Coping Resources to Occupational Stress and Strain*, 32:1 J. VOCATIONAL BEHAVIOR 1–15 (1988).

38. S.H. OSIPOW, OCCUPATIONAL STRESS INVENTORY 2, 13 (rev. ed. 1998).

39. S.L. Kirmeyer & T.W. Dougherty, *Work Load, Tension, and Coping: Moderating Effects of Supervisor Support*, 41:2 PERSONNEL PSYCHOL. 125–39 (1988).

40. D. Munz et al., *A Worksite Stress Management Program: Theory, Application, and Outcomes, in* JOB STRESS INTERVENTIONS 57–72 (L.R. Murphy et al. eds., 1995).

41. R.S. LAZARUS & S. FOLKMAN, STRESS APPRAISAL AND COPING (1984).

42. D.D. BURNS, THE FEELING GOOD HANDBOOK (1989).

43. M. SELIGMAN, LEARNED OPTIMISM (1991).

44. S.R. Maddi et al., *The Effectiveness of Hardiness Training*, 50:2 CONSULTING PSYCHOL. J.: PRAC. & RES. 78–86 (1998).

45. D. Ganster, *Interventions for Building Healthy Organizations: Suggestions from the Stress Research Literature, in* JOB STRESS INTERVENTIONS 323–36 (L.R. Murphy et al. eds., 1995).

46. M. Peterson, *Work, Corporate Culture, and Stress: Implications for Worksite Health Promotion*, 21:4 AM. J. HEALTH BEHAVIOR 243–52 (1997).

47. T.A. Beehr & J.E. Newman, *Job Stress, Employee Health and Organizational Effectiveness: A Facet Analysis, Model and Literature Review*, 31:6 PERSONNEL PSYCHOL. 665–99 (1978).

48. M. WEINSTEIN, MANAGING TO HAVE FUN (1996).

49. J.M. Ivancevich et al., *Worksite Stress Management Interventions*, 45 AMERICAN PSYCHOLOGIST 252–61 (1990).

50. D.D. BURNS, THE FEELING GOOD HANDBOOK (1989).

51. M. SELIGMAN, LEARNED OPTIMISM (1991).

52. J. Hurell & L. Murphy, *An Overview of Occupational Stress and Health, in* ENVIRONMENTAL AND OCCUPATIONAL MEDICINE, SECOND EDITION 675–84 (W.M. Rom ed., 1992).

53. D.C. Ganster & J. Schaubroeck, *Work Stress and Employee Health*, 17:4 J. OF MGMT. 235–71 (1991).

54. M.R. Manning et al., *Occupational Stress and Health Care Use*, 1:1 J. OCCUPATIONAL HEALTH PSYCHOL. 100–09 (1996).

55. S. Cartwright et al., *Diagnosing a Healthy Organization: A Proactive Approach to Stress in the Workplace, in* JOB STRESS INTERVENTIONS 217–34 (L.R. Murphy et al. eds., 1995).

56. D. Ganster, *Interventions for Building Healthy Organizations: Suggestions from the Stress Research Literature, in* JOB STRESS INTERVENTIONS 323–36 (L.R. Murphy et al. eds., 1995).

CHAPTER 11

Taming the Rhinoceros: Getting, Maintaining, and Wielding Power for Corporate Ethics and Compliance

Mary Ann Bowman Beil

Power is a delegated right or privilege to compel obedience by one who has influence. It poses one of the most significant professional dilemmas for the corporate ethics and compliance officer (CECO). Power attends the role and the responsibilities of the CECO, but CECOs face a challenge in attaining power and then exercising that power often with virtually no executive authority. This fact alone distinguishes the demands on the talents and skills of the CECO in a way that is unmatched and often misunderstood by other members of the senior management team.

There is a story about the time that the authors Alexander Woollcott and G. K. Chesterton met for lunch at a London restaurant.[1] Chesterton, not surprisingly, was expounding on a wide range of philosophical topics when he began to talk about the relationship between power and authority. "If a rhinoceros were to enter this restaurant now, there is no denying he would have great power here. But I should be the first to rise and assure him that he had no authority whatever."

In many ways, every CECO appears like a rhinoceros on the horizon of his or her institution. Others in the organization may think the CECO possesses substantive power when, in fact, the CECO does not have clearly defined authority. There is a fragile balance between power and authority, especially for the CECO who focuses specifically on the skills and techniques that can be implemented in order to enhance power—or, in the absence of power, effectiveness. CECOs acquire power primarily from three different sources: (1) formal authority, (2) chief executive officer (CEO) empowerment, and (3) personal moral authority. Moreover, how they exercise that power depends, in part, on how and when an organization

217

chooses to hire them. The CECO's ability to function effectively will depend on how artfully he or she can weave together the elements of power and authority that are available to him or her at any given time. The first two sources of power—formal authority and CEO empowerment—are primarily external and subject to greater variation. The third source of power—personal moral authority—is a function of the CECO's own character and ability to provide the still waters required to navigate safely the increasingly treacherous regulatory topography of health care.

As a new role in the health care industry, there is little precedence for how an organization should empower the position of CECO. The office does not come with a single imprimatur of power. In fact, there is no single—much less, well-trodden—path to the corporate ethics and compliance office. The way that organizations designate a corporate ethics and compliance officer differs markedly from CECO to CECO. Some organizations select their CECO internally by asking someone to move into the role. Increasingly, organizations are hiring someone from the outside to serve in the role. Moreover, some organizations hire a CECO under the requirements of a Corporate Integrity Agreement, while other organizations hire a CECO in an effort to avoid the same. Some CEOs hire a CECO, while other CEOs inherit their CECO. Finally, some CECOs will work for private not-for-profit health care systems, for-profit health systems, or for any combination of ownership-management arrangement between the two.

This list of possibilities is merely to show the variety of management scenarios that will influence the power and authority of any particular CECO at any give time in the life of an organization. There is no one standard for power and authority; and, as far as is apparent, there is no continuum along which the two can be charted and monitored for progress. It is actually a bit more like a high-tech stock in the first two quarters of 2000—unpredictable, and up and down. In the case of one organization, it hired a CECO in the midst of a public relations fiasco resulting from a schism between the board, management, and medical staff that exposed misconduct. Thus, the position was initiated with the full support of the board and the then interim CEO.

An institution's board—guided by the Federal Sentencing Commission and inspired by the enforcement efforts of the Department of Health and Human Services (HHS)—ought officially to delegate authority to a CECO. However, the CEO will ultimately determine what power, if any, the corporate CECO will have in the institution. The working relationship between CEO and CECO is crucial, therefore, in determining the power of the CECO.

Some may question why it is assumed here that the CECO reports directly to the CEO, when that may not be the case. Similarly, some may suggest that perhaps the CECO should report directly to the board of directors. It is agreed that the CECO should have the kind of open and candid communication with the board that is appropriate for the role. However, it could be argued that the CECO should report administratively directly to the CEO and not the board. The art of compliance depends on a creative debate between the CECO and the CEO. Together, the CECO and the CEO must determine which issues are a matter of governance and which issues disclose a pattern of compliance risks that must be reported to the board. The art of compliance requires a high level of trust between the CECO and the CEO. It may be difficult to achieve this level of trust, but without the CEO's trust the CECO will not acquire the power necessary to do the job.

Trustworthiness, then, is the most important quality for the CECO. Trust is the foundation of the power that the officer may acquire from time to time. Although a simple concept, trust is difficult to achieve in real institutional life. The foundations of a trusting relationship have a lot to do with the appointment of the CECO. If a CEO handpicks the CECO, then the CECO has the best opportunity to build a trusting relationship with that CEO. In fact, the best opportunity exists for a trusting relationship when the CEO exercises an option to select a long-trusted colleague from the management ranks. When this is the case, the road to trust, to power, and then to influence is already two-thirds traveled.

Finally, in some cases, a new CEO inherits an incumbent CECO. This may well be the most challenging match for both executives. Management styles are unknown, problem-resolution techniques are unknown, and the basic values by which each responds to an issue are untested. Essentially the CECO is starting over. CECOs err when they assume that they can maintain under a new administration the power that they acquired under a previous administration. CECOs should assume that only the personal stuff of character and credibility survives the transition from one CEO to another.

Whether an organization hires a CECO by internal selection, or by external hire, or a new CEO inherits a CECO, this initial relationship will be the starting point for discovering or, more accurately, unraveling the aspects and origins of the CECO's power. Regardless of the common threads that establish the authority of the position—the Federal Sentencing Guidelines, institutional board charters, Office of Inspector General (OIG) Advisories, or settlement agreements—the power of the position will emerge subtly and will be less clearly defined.

The external factors that provide much of the formal authority for the CECO are important and valuable. In combination with the institutional landscape, external factors also serve as the starting point of empowerment. If an organization hires a CECO to satisfy requirements of a settlement agreement, or to address serious and potentially expensive compliance issues, or to address business conduct issues in the aftermath or midst of a public relations fiasco, the CECO will more often than not begin his or her tenure in a stronger position to acquire and execute power. This is not surprising, as management perceives the CECO to be part of the solution to a problem that clearly threatens the institution. It is in the best interests of the CEO and the board to empower the CECO and to sustain that power. Under these circumstances, the CECO has the most difficult starting point, but often begins in the strongest position from which to proceed.

One cannot predict whether the CECO will be able to sustain this level of power through an initial critical moment. Experience has proven that the CECO often cannot sustain it. For this reason, an analysis of the basis of a CECO's power is far more complex than the executive power of senior management. The function of CECO calls for power sufficient to influence the institution. However, absent executive authority, the CECO must rely on the CEO, the board, moral authority, and the force of character.

Empowerment by the CEO is the single most important factor in determining what power the CECO is perceived to have in his or her role on a day-to-day basis. When this empowerment is apparent, consistent, and bestowed on the competent officer, the CECO realizes sufficient power to be truly effective. Of course, the CECO may not be ineffective in the absence of this empowerment, but he or she will be faced with a far more difficult task in getting the job done.

This concept of "empowerment" is so important that it is absolutely necessary to understand how it appears in reality, beyond semantics and contemporary business lingo. It is an almost overused term in business today, but the CECO and the CEO need to know precisely what "empowerment" looks and sounds like in the context of this particular discussion. Graydon Wood, the former Vice-President of Corporate Ethics and Business Conduct at NYNEX, succinctly clarified this issue during a transition in leadership. Graydon argued that the CEO will determine the level of power and, ultimately, influence that the CECO will have by what he or she says publicly. If, in management and leadership meetings, the CEO says things like "I'd like our corporate ethics and compliance officer to look at that question" or, deferring to the CECO in a meeting, asks, "What do you think about this particular issue?" or, in responding to another senior-level executive, says, "I'd like you to have a discussion with the CECO before we make a final decision," or "I'd like you to send that document to the CECO before we sign off on it," then the signs are posted that the CEO is empowering the CECO in his or her position. It is a message that every member of the senior management team hears clearly, and it carries far more weight than any title the officer may have or any official meetings in which he or she may be included. Nothing else compares to the CEO publicly handing the mantle to the CECO.

A CECO is either the beneficiary of this level of empowerment or not. There is no room for "in-between" on this score. Either the CEO makes it clear that the CECO has the power to work with management toward the ends that the leadership has mutually defined, or the CECO faces the stark reality of an uphill climb. A favorite metaphor for what it is like to be a CECO comes from a sport—alpine-style mountain climbing. The climber learns to self-arrest (a lifesaving technique used to stop one's uncontrolled fall) and to use fixed lines in order to summit. The metaphor of the "fixed lines" best describes what it is like to do compliance work in the presence of clear empowerment. The highest and most frequently attempted summits in the world have established base camps for frequent climbers and expeditions. As the expeditions reach the highest and most treacherous faces of the climb, they will find fixed lines, which are simply ropes anchored to the route by experienced climbers who preceded them. If he or she chooses, the CEO can anchor those fixed lines for the CECO as well as for the rest of the expedition or leadership team.

More important, perhaps, than making the role of CECO easier, the CEO has a vested interest in openly and enthusiastically choosing to empower the CECO. The credit for this insight goes to Craig Drielinger, President of the Drielinger Group, who posed a simple clarifying question in one of his seminars that every CECO should be required to ask annually. "When is the last time that you asked your CEO how the work that you were doing in corporate ethics and compliance could further the CEO's goals?" It is an exquisite question. Even with strategic plans, benchmarking, operational goals, and routine performance reports, few CECOs have probably asked that question. Do this one thing tomorrow, because you will be surprised at the answer—or lack of one. When the CECO can effectively align—and one should not assume that they are aligned —with the real goals of the CEO, there is a far better opportunity for empowerment because it is in the CEO's self-interest. (As an aside, it is recommended that this question be posed individually to every member of the senior management team because it will provide the CECO with a body of valuable information on which to build future compliance plans, organization direction for corporate ethics and compliance, and working relationships.)

As suggested earlier, a CECO knows when he or she is not empowered by the CEO. Even if the CEO values the CECO and his or her role on the management team, it is not the same as publicly empowering him or her. That is why it is possible to find scenarios where a CEO may like, admire, and respect the person in the compliance role, but still does not empower him or her; and vice versa, where a CEO does not personally like the person in the role, but may empower him or her to get the job done. And of course, some CEOs just do not know how to empower publicly. It sounds incredible, but it is a fact in spite of being one inconsistent with the qualities that are usually expected in chief executives. In that case, forgive the CEO the shortcoming, teach him or her, but get on with the task at hand, knowing that "power" and subsequently "effectiveness" will be a bit more challenging. The CECO need not be daunted. The job can still get done.

The CECO's sources of power are two parts external—authority and CEO empowerment—and one part internal—character. External sources of power will most likely vary throughout the tenure of the CECO; they will wax and wane, impacted by the regulatory environment, board commitments, management changes, and the vagaries of corporate and industry politics. The CECO may not have control over external sources of power, but it just makes sense for the CECO continually to monitor and know at what level each of these external sources of power is in play at any given time so that the officer can strategically negotiate the peaks and valleys of empowerment in a manner that will be less damaging to the effectiveness of the role.

The third and final source of power is personal. It is the CECO's most important source of power, and the only source of power entirely under the CECO's control. The third source of power can exist and provide the essential elements of effectiveness in the absence of the other two external sources of power. Conversely, in the absence of this particular personal source of power, the other two are meaningless. Personal power does not wax and wane; it expands exponentially with experience, competence, and the ability to survive occasional institutional travail.

Every CECO knows the foundations on which he or she has forged his or her character and moral strength. CECOs are tapped most often for their credibility, trustworthiness, strength, independence, and diplomacy, in addition to their competencies. It is a certain force of character that enhances the CECO's effectiveness and strengthens the overall cultural fabric of the institution. This force of character and source of power require the CECO's attention professionally as well personally. In other senior executive roles, character is certainly an asset, but in the corporate ethics and compliance role it is the substance. As the substance and the only sure power that goes hand in hand with the job, it is to be nurtured, protected, and developed.

One of the most baffling challenges in the profession of corporate ethics and compliance is determining where the officer fits in the institutional structure. It can be daunting just figuring out what the day-to-day tasks of achieving corporate ethics and compliance are once the CECO moves beyond the U.S. Sentencing Guidelines. Because many CECOs emerge from the ranks of line management, they are challenged when exploring how to influence the operational life of the institution without muddying up the works. The CECO ponders how to "do something" to prove that the office is worth the institution's investment. I struggled with this issue off and on the first year. Candidly, power was the last thing on my mind as I struggled with the more remedial concern of what one does when appointed the CECO.

About a year into my tenure, a consultant appeared who was assessing institutional operations as part of a management transition. The consultant was Cy Hufano, now vice president of Cap Gemini Ernst & Young. Corporate ethics and compliance was not on his operational radar screen during the engagement, but he generously conceded to review the structure and foundations upon which the institution's corporate ethics and compliance program was taking shape. At the conclusion of the presentation to him, Cy said that he found what I had presented to him to be an interesting model, highly integrated and potentially effective. He then turned, looked directly at me, and continued saying that he could not understand why someone who appeared to care so deeply about the organization would function in a way that could so seriously weaken its management structure.

What did Cy Hufano mean? He meant—and, I might add, he had "nailed it" perfectly—that because I was not clear on what was operationally appropriate for the role, I was (even though well meaning) propping up weaknesses in line management by doing the work in the line, then stepping back out. What he helped me to see is how important it is to be restrained as a CECO. It is better to advise, assist, monitor, and recommend required changes. This would be the only way in which the corporate ethics and compliance role would be an appropriate part of senior management. It would also be the only way truly to achieve the integrated model of ethics and compliance that I had designed and aspired to see in operational reality.

The reason that I mention this story in the context of personal power is because I had to enhance personal resources—particularly self-confidence and restraint—in order to change the way I was doing the job. Restraint was perhaps the most important quality. Shortly after this revelatory discussion, I tried to figure out a way to explain to employees how the corporate ethics and compliance office and officer worked, and then I asked an artist to illustrate my concept. The illustration is an exploding tapestry ball that surrounds a spiked ball in the center. The tapestry fabric that shields the spiked structure is made up of many different colored threads that represent the multiple compliance competencies that are required throughout the health care system. Virtually every position in the system requires some compliance competency and strength. It may be a competency in Joint Commission on Accreditation of Healthcare Organizations requirements, credentialing, Occupational Safety and Health Administration (OSHA), the Employee Retirement Income Security Act (ERISA), the Health Care Financing Administration (HCFA), the Department of Insurance, or accreditation—the list goes on. How effectively the company is managed determines the pattern in the fabric and how well woven those compliance competencies are at any given time. Finally, the opportunities for ethical development within the institution are important independent of compliance. The four concentric and expanding layers that extend beyond the tapestry ball demonstrate those opportunities. Those layers represent the four stages of ethical development outlined in Driscoll, Hoffmann, and Petry's text, *The Ethical Edge:*[2] (1) ethical awareness, (2) ethical training, (3) ethical action, and (4) ethical leadership.

CECOs, particularly the ones who strive to posit the institution's corporate compliance program in the broader context of a corporate ethics initiative, depend significantly on personal power to respond to the messages that alert the institution to a weakened or threatened fabric. The mission to move individuals, departments, divisions, and whole institutions toward ethical leadership demands that the CECO has power that is competently applied.

It is of value from time to time to stop and graph where, as the CECO, to place senior managers, team leaders, departments, and employees on this topography. This exercise results in a clear image of where the officer's actions and energies should be directed for individual and collective improvement in compliance. Of the books that inspire the CECO in his or her work, there is one that should be required reading. Gordon MacKenzie's *Orbiting the Giant Hairball (A Corporate Fool's Guide to Surviving with Grace)*[3] is a book that explores the ways any executive might inspire institutional change, and even transformation. With humor, insight, a pinch of corporate cynicism, and a hilarious view of bureaucracy, MacKenzie guides the reader to the options outside the hairball while warning of the ineffectiveness that can occur when one moves completely out of orbit. MacKenzie's book should be required reading for those officers who struggle with where and how the CECO fits in the management structure. The CECO who functions outside of traditional line operations, but who is still expected to influence the entire institution toward enhanced compliance, ethics, and performance, will discover fun and unconventional methods to get job done. It is a survival guide when the CECO senses that his or her power—not to mention passion and enthusiasm—are on the wane.

Sometimes the only power available to the CECO is to provide a breath of inspiration to the front line employee, middle manager, or leader who is at the end of his or her rope in an industry that has been burdened with ever-expanding regulatory requirements, rapidly shrinking reimbursement for essential health services, and the stretching of staff to provide those services—all of which is to be accomplished without threatening the quality of care. In an industry that deals with human life and health, there is nothing more difficult than knowing that the margin for error—in care and compliance—may be narrowing every day. It is a fact that every CECO must acknowledge and, on a day-to-day basis, deal with in his or her work. For this reason, the concept of servant leadership that was introduced initially in two essays by Robert Greenleaf[4] in the 1970s is such a valid leadership model for the CECO today. Servant leadership is the belief that one is only as important or equipped to lead those whom one is to serve. Thus, the higher one rises in an institution, the deeper his or her commitment to serve those whom he or she is to guide. Thinking in these terms as the CECO, this concept translates to serving the entire institution, its business partners, customers, and community. It is a servant position, but it is in that servanthood that the officer's real power emerges.

There are days when the CECO is banging his or her head against the corporate wall. There are other days when the CECO is convinced that he or she never did have any power—or, if he or she did have power, it is now lost. On those days, one struggling team member experiencing the CECO's commitment to a servant style of leadership will carry the officer through to fight another day. More important, it is at this moment, when the concept of power is completely devoid of ego and when the officer is most vulnerable, that he or she will experience the grace that can be bestowed only by the one being served. Unlike the empowerment by the CEO, which may or may not be there from time to time, the empowerment of the servant leader by the beneficiary of his or her service is almost always assured. It is this empowerment of the servant by those that are served that keeps full the CECO's coffers of professional energy, passion, and influence.

Finally, and continuing with the argument that the third source of power—personal—is the most compelling, there is one question that occurs to every CECO at least once—if not once a day—in his or her tenure: Can the CECO lead without power? Although the question is adapted to a specific management role in an organization, the question emerges from the title and thesis of Max De Pree's book, *Leading without Power: Finding Hope in Serving Community*.[5] The book speaks to not-for-profit institutions and the lessons that they may provide to for-profits in leadership and commitment to purpose. De Pree's book resonates with health care institutions because whether one is the CECO in a for-profit system, provider, or insurer; in a not-for-profit serving single or multiple communities; or in a not-for-profit managed by a for-profit health care company, the institution is an "agency of care." More important, the employees in health care institutions are there precisely because they are drawn—some would say called—to lives of service. In De Pree's words, "moral purpose and active virtue" drive them.

"Without moral purpose, competence has no measure and trust no goal."[6] For Max De Pree, that clear moral purpose in life results in active virtue. It is creating and maintaining a landscape upon which employees can exercise this active virtue that is one of the most important reasons for the CECO to claim and execute power and influence whenever possible. When the CECO is convinced that there is insufficient power in the role, then this is when the employees—moving in active virtue with the wind of moral purpose in their sails—will move across the institutional landscape to further the ethics and compliance goals.

Almost two decades ago, when I was living in Atlanta, I had a friend who was an accomplished long-distance runner. He and others who could run these impressive distances belonged to a group called the "Hashers." One Saturday every month, my friend would wake up in the wee hours of the morning and, with a can of brightly colored spray paint, set out to run the day's entire route, stopping at each point of departure to paint a bright arrow on the road or tree to mark the path for the runners who would begin the race at a designated starting point later that morning. I have often thought that the role of the CECO was not unlike that of the "hasher" who would wake up in the early hours to paint the arrows on the path and then return to run in the pack. Perhaps it is not power that the CECO needs to be effective, but rather the ability to get up early, have plenty of cans of paint, and the ability to hold our own with the pack.

Chesterton was not far off the mark in his debate with Woollcott. The CECO probably does arrive on the institutional scene a bit like the rhinoceros in the restaurant. And, like the rhinoceros, it is wise always to be aware of how daunting and dangerous that power—when all three sources are in full supply—can appear to observers. With the full power of external authority, the public empowerment of the CEO, and the personal power of the individual, a CECO could well wield it all in a manner that could destroy the restaurant and ruin everyone's meal. That is why the more sources of power that one is able to marshal to the cause at any given time, the more important it is to understand its measure and impact.

To exercise power with the appropriate measure of strength or gentleness as the issue may require becomes the single ability that distinguishes the compliance professional who exercises power as an art form instead of a heavy-handed management technique. The artful rhinoceros will somehow find a place in the institution, in the boardroom, and at the senior management table, and will find some way to get the job done. And on the days when the rhinoceros is feeling powerless and sits absolutely silent, everyone in the company will certainly know that the rhinoceros is still there.

NOTES

1. G.K. Chesterton, Charles Dickens: The Last of the Great Men Foreword x (1942).

2. Dawn-Marie Driscoll et al., The Ethical Edge: Tales of Organizations That Have Faced Moral Crisis 185 (1995).

3. G. MacKenzie, Orbiting The Giant Hairball (A Corporate Fool's Guide to Surviving with Grace) 40–41 (1998).

4. R.K. Greenleaf, Servant Leadership: A Journey Into the Nature of Legitimate Power and Greatness 7–48 (1977).

5. M. De Pree, Leading Without Power: Finding Hope in Serving Community 179–86 (1997).

6. M. De Pree, Leading Without Power: Finding Hope in Serving Community (1997).

CHAPTER 12

The Nimble Professional: Developing and Polishing Career Skills

Felicia McAleer

INTRODUCTION

The "nimble professional"[1] can be found in any walk of life or industry. Undoubtedly, there are many such professionals in the field of compliance. They are easily recognized as they are sought after by professional associations, recruiters, publishers, and the best companies and organizations. They seem to breeze through life with a steady stream of career opportunities. They seem to manage easily their professional responsibilities and balance them with a rewarding family and social life. They are often found serving their community by sitting on the board of the ballet or leading a team to build the next house for groups like Habit for Humanity. They are fit, energetic, never too busy to help, and return communications (e-mail, telephone calls, or faxes) almost immediately. Executive managers seek out their ideas and opinions, and their employees and colleagues enjoy working with them.

Webster's definition of *nimble* is quick to understand, think, and devise.[2] Nimble professionals demonstrate these skills as they make sound decisions quickly and have a track record to substantiate their judgments. They are outgoing, but never monopolize a conversation. They are flexible, but not compromising on critical issues where their persuasive abilities can win out. They have a sense of urgency, but do not appear to be overly stressed. They are sensitive and empathetic, but never seem overwhelmed by their emotions. They respect others and make people feel special. They adhere to policies and also suggest new possibilities. They lead by example and do not demand respect; they earn it!

Who and where are nimble professionals? They are everywhere. You could be one now or could grow to be such a professional. John Lucht, in *The New Rites of Passage at $100,000+,* states that an interviewer hopes to find the following attributes in a candidate. These attributes are borrowed to describe the nimble professional:

> Intelligent, and also "street smart," with abundant common sense. Analytical, logical, goal-oriented, and a planner. A skilled communicator . . . good at listening, speaking, and writing. Unmistakably a leader . . . but also a "team player," cooperative, and congenial. Healthful, attractive, and well groomed. Tasteful in dress and decorum. Poised, courteous, and cultured. Sensitive to the feelings of others . . . not pushy, pig-headed, or obnoxious. Honest, loyal, and straightforward. Politically aware, but not a political operator. Committed, responsible, and diligent. Cheerful and optimistic, with a "can do" attitude. And overall, an interesting person, with curiosity, enthusiasm . . . and maybe even a sense of humor![3]

Attributes from Stephen Covey's *Principle-Centered Leadership* are also borrowed to describe nimble professionals: "They are continually learning; service oriented; radiate positive energy; believe in other people; lead balanced lives; see life as an adventure; are continually synergistic; and exercise for self-renewal."[4] Nimble professionals also recognize the four dimensions of human personality—physical, mental, emotional, and spiritual—and they understand how to work with these different components in themselves and others.

Measure yourself against these attributes. If you fall short, develop methods and processes in your career and professional development to enhance the quality of your life and the lives of those who surround you. For the already successful professional, the purposes of this chapter are to assure you that you are on the right track and to offer some ideas on expanding and enhancing your plans and contributions. For those of you who have no plan, essentially no networking contacts, and are virtually unknown in your field, the chapter offers some suggestions to prepare for a better future. What follows is a consolidation of the best tips and advice from career planners, image consultants, recruiting and executive search professionals, financial experts, résumé writers, and interview coaches.

THE NIMBLE CAREER PLAN

There are few "right place, right time" opportunities in real life. Opportunities tend to be created by those who have planned well, and are prepared and packaged properly. Nimble professionals know that planning, preparing, and creating a package is not a one-time event; it is a lifestyle. They have not only one plan, but several contingency plans that create flexibility and options for their future.

Most professionals recognize the necessity of ongoing educational, technical, and interpersonal skills development, but often see their hopes for advancement disappear because their skills, abilities, and potential lack the proper planning and preparation in critical areas, such as creating an "Image Package" and a solid "Financial Foundation." Both of these are so important that they have their own section below.

Creating a plan, finding the right organization, and creating the proper package to ensure that you are being well represented sounds simple. Of course, the difficulty is in the implementation. Several compliance professionals have commented on the difficulty of developing a career plan in an emerging field where established career paths do not exist. Degree programs, certifications, or even role models for the field are just being developed. On the other hand, emerging fields offer an opportunity for you to design the profession, as well as your own career.

How does one plan for emerging careers? Stephen Covey suggests that one should, "Begin with the end in mind."[5] This means that you should build a career plan (and even a life plan) based on what you want to achieve and the results you want to create. Do not get hung up in having the *right* answer, as there is no such thing. This is a discovery process and it may take some time to decide how you want your life and career to progress.

You might begin by writing the story of your retirement. Create a retirement party scenario of you at your best, including the results of all the planning and enhancing you are going to do over the next decade or so. What age are you? Who is there? What have you accomplished financially in your life and career? How is your health? What are your plans after retirement? What foundation have you created to provide for your financial freedom? What were you known for in your industry? What contributions did you make that made a difference in your industry, family, community, and the world? How have you remained flexible and open to opportunities and able to "see" the opportunities that other people miss?

Now write your funeral eulogy. Many people find this exercise emotionally upsetting, but everyone is, after all, mortal, and each life will one day be a story told. So, try it as an exercise. Write the things for which you want to be remembered. List all your friends and loved ones who have come to say goodbye. Is anyone missing? Are there any relationships that you need to mend to complete the guest list? What did you fail to accomplish? What apologies needed to be made? This exercise may provide the incentive to begin making changes that will enhance the rest of your life.

Most professionals spend more time planning their next vacation than the two critical components of their life, their career and their financial foundation. Of course the two are usually linked, unless you win the lottery. Without a plan with many contingencies built into it, people often wake up middle aged and ask, "Who am I and how did I get here?" Once a client in a career life-planning workshop said, "Oh, I forgot to have children." But there was a ring of truth and sadness in this confession. Another client offered, "It will soon be time for me to retire and I don't have enough money." The typical excuses for not planning are that people do not have time, do not believe that a plan will work in any case, or do not know how to develop and stick to a plan. But it is true that they had better make the time or time will make them. Some people say that they do not believe in planning because they believe that a plan does not guarantee success. It is true that having a plan does not guarantee success. However, they also admit that attempting to create a plan caused them to consider important issues like: what they want out of life and a career, how might they get there, what they will do if they do not get there, how many roads lead there, who can help them to get there, what skills and tools will they need to get there, and what they will do if they get there and do not like it. Many compliance professionals have expressed that they have experienced limited growth opportunities, which some have attributed to lack of careful career planning and networking.

Most people develop the skills to plan a vacation, build an addition to their home, get an education, put together a party, or complete many successful projects at work. Those same project design, planning, management, and implementation techniques and skills will help you create the flexible plan needed to become "the nimble professional."

THE NIMBLE JOB SEARCH

Nimble professionals are always prepared for a job search. One never knows when the next job search may be necessary, or under what circumstances, so prepare now. Get everything in order—résumé, interview skills, networking contacts, financial foundation, emergency job search plan, image audit—and be prepared.

But before discussing the job search, think about what you would do if you lost your job today. This could easily happen in the compliance field. What would you do if you lost your job and foresaw no immediate prospects for a new job? For most people, sudden job loss is a worst-case scenario. You can better manage the process by understanding the emotional forces at work by having the above-discussed plan in place. But many people have admitted that before they could move forward with a new job search, they first had to deal with the stress, anxiety, and anger created by losing their job and by their fear of the future.

The first reaction to losing your job may be panic. One man hid this reaction from his family and friends, with a disastrous outcome. Some people even go to the extreme of leaving home every day as if they were going to their job. Avoid the temptation to panic and deceive. Family and friends can provide enormous support and make it easier for you to proceed with a successful job search.

> After the initial panic has subsided, you may begin to blame yourself for your plight. You may feel that you have let yourself and your family down, or be convinced that job prospects are going to be pretty poor. Obviously, these feelings are not going to help your situation, but you need to recognize that you are likely to go through this stage. Finally, you will begin to feel angry about your situation. It is not until you get through this last stage that you will be in the frame of mind to present yourself to a prospective employer convincingly. This stage typically leads to renewed self-confidence and determination.[6]

To prepare for your unemployed time, start and continue a daily routine of exercise and stress management. Your doctor should be consulted before starting a new program. Consider community service work to take your mind off your problems and to contribute to others in need. Take advantage of any career outplacement or counseling services that your company offers or seek assistance on your own with a professional who has a successful track record. Cut expenses and seek methods of creating additional income using special talents that you may have such as writing, tutoring, building furniture, or landscaping. Contact your "network," which should include industry recruiters, and get to work. Getting a job *is* a job! "Take advantage of unemployment compensation to which you are entitled (or can negotiate) and continue or replace the all-important em-ployer-provided health insurance coverage."[7] "[Try to] keep up with your mortgage payments, since your house is probably your largest investment. [Unless you are the exception], resist the temptation that many laid-off people have of starting their own business. [And, if] it appears likely that you are going to have trouble meeting your obligations to creditors, be sure to contact them and work out a more comfortable payment schedule."[8]

As personally devastating as being laid off or dismissed from a job can be, an even move difficult situation could develop if you encounter an ethi-cal conflict while employed that warrants your resignation. Plan for this contingency as well. Do some research to discover what legal rights you have if you were asked to make some unethical decisions or look the other way concerning illegal activities on your job. Do you understand what is illegal, and what may be arguably legal but unethical? What could cause you to compromise your integrity? What legal protection do you have if you report illegal or unethical activities? What statute of limitation laws apply that regulate your industry? Who are the top attorneys in your field? What "whistle-blower" laws apply? What steps would you take internally and externally to resolve an issue like this?

When you are ready to begin your job search, you should know that job searches fall into two general categories: (1) specific, customized searches in which you contact only a few companies, and (2) broad searches in which you contact many firms from several industries. Regardless of the strategy you employ, your approach should be similar to designing a mar-keting project. You must develop leads, mail documents, set up a filing system for follow-up calls, and prepare your sales presentation, interview, and telemarketing scripts.

You will need to monitor all contacts and mail for follow-up, manage files for easy reference, and prepare the home telephone system to present a professional image to a caller. Children are adorable and wonderful, but they should not be answering the telephone when you are doing a job search. A rude spouse or roommate also should not be a part of your incoming call management system. A busy recruiter said that, after making hundreds of calls, they were not amused by a rude spouse or children who could not take a message, and moved that résumé to the bottom of the pile. Answering machine messages should reflect your professionalism, not your playfulness. Many professionals put only their cell phone number on their résumé to ensure proper call handling.

Your job search now has a new weapon, the Internet. Job hunters today research job opportunities and target companies through the Internet before launching their job search. This approach is a new one that may well help you gain an edge over your competition in finding new leads and researching companies before an interview. Recruiters are also a great source of job opportunities. There are basically two types of recruiters: retained and contingency. Retained search professionals contract for specific searches and contingency recruiters have job openings, but not necessarily a contract or an exclusive agreement with the hiring company. Typically, executives seek retained search professionals, but you may find occasion to work with a contingency recruiter if there is a legitimate listing and it is from a company that you would not have contacted if the contingency recruiter had not persuaded you. Often managing your job search without a recruiter is the best way to go, especially if you have contacts within a company with which you wish to work. You may be better off without a recruiting fee attached to your hire. However, remember that recruiters of either type typically work for their client company, not for you. Nevertheless, if you market yourself properly to search professionals and maintain a relationship with recruiters in your industry, they can be a great resource for job opportunities and sometimes career direction. You help create a relationship when you send them an updated résumé, give them leads of potential candidates when you are not qualified, and, whenever possible, use their services to hire for your company.

You will need a good set of references that can be provided with your résumé, or you may announce on your résumé that references will be submitted upon request. Call those who are providing your references and prepare them with specific job descriptions. Refresh their memory of critical areas to cover. You might send them notes to refresh their memory, as well. Take them to lunch, if possible, and rekindle the relationship. Be sure to thank them for their assistance now and after you get the job.

Also, consider the situation where the timing is right to conduct a job search while you are still employed. Obviously, you will tell your interviewers not to contact your current employer while you are looking and you will need to provide references who will keep your search confidential. Perhaps someone who knew you in your current job but has left your company would be a good reference. This situation also brings the issues of resigning and counter offers into the job search process.

Once you decide to accept an offer, you can accept it verbally but realize that, until you have the offer in writing, you do not have a firm offer. Once you receive the offer in writing, write a resignation letter stating simply that you are resigning, noting your last day of employment, and hand it to your boss. It is not recommended that you go into great detail about your new job or why you are leaving. Burning bridges does you no good. Handle your acceptance, counter offers, and resignation as a professional. Leave doors open whenever possible. You may receive a counter offer from your current firm if you are still employed, but be careful. Your peers and even the manager and company that make the counter offer may think that you obtained the counter offer through coercion (that is, by threatening to quit). Accepting a counter offer seldom works as you have now alienated both companies to a certain extent, as well as your recruiter and networking contacts who referred you. It is often better to negotiate a good offer and stick with it. Notify other companies, recruiters, and your references that you have found a job and would like to keep in contact with them for the future. Remember to keep records of job search expenses to discuss with your accountant.

NIMBLE CAREER AND PROFESSIONAL DEVELOPMENT

Nimble career and professional development includes, ideally, a lifetime commitment to continuing education, personal development, maximizing networking opportunities, creating an impeccable reputation, and becoming an industry leader. It will be easier when you create and follow a plan. The development plan needs to include enhancing or neutralizing your own sabotaging behaviors, mastering advanced communications, and becoming a credible leader. Getting ahead will depend a great deal on your ability to supervise, manage, and lead people. You will often need to lead a team or serve on a committee with people you do not actually manage or over whom you have no authority. The first thing you need to think about when managing people are the differences between acting as a manager, director, dictator, coach, and leader. In different situations, and with different people, each style could be appropriate. Leaders are not born; they are created. You cannot demand respect and loyalty; you must earn it.

Try this exercise as part of your professional development plan. Write down the qualities and attributes that you think a great leader should or could have. What leader have you followed and what positive attributes did he or she have? How many of these qualities do you have? What can or will you do to achieve these skills, qualities, and attributes? What behaviors will you need to modify and under what circumstances? Remember that awareness of what you need to do is a good first step. However, significant change may require help. You will need a plan and a method to measure yourself as you change behaviors and you may want to ask for honest feedback from peers, team members, your manager, and those you love, and then modify your behavior accordingly.

Managers and leaders also need to understand how to manage *power*. Certain types of mishandled power and inappropriate control create fear, stifle creativity, diminish trust, and destroy loyalty for the leader and the company. Stephen Covey recommends what he calls *legitimate power*:

> Legitimate power is based on the power people have because others tend to believe in them and in what they are trying to accomplish. Legitimate power leaders are trusted, respected, and honored. And they are followed because others want to follow them. Legitimate power is rare. It is sustained because it is not dependent on whether or not something desirable or undesirable happens to the follower. It is created when the values of the followers and the values of the leader overlap. Legitimate power is not forced. Control is apparent with legitimate power, but the control is not external; it is self-control.[9]

Also, many savvy professionals have developed an internal and external public relations campaign as part of their career and professional development plan; they are the first ones to be called for job opportunities and industry conferences. These nimble professionals find themselves at the right place, at the right time, with the right package and the right contacts. It means going a step beyond typical networking by becoming known inside your company and throughout your industry for your expertise, leadership, and integrity. It means clearly understanding the expectations others have of you and exceeding those expectations. This means mentoring and coaching others. It includes getting involved with professional associations, not only by conference attendance, but also by service on boards and committees. It means organizing and hosting conferences and meetings, public speaking, and writing for the trade publications. The following three organizations are recommended for compliance professionals in the health care industry: (1) the Health Care Compliance Association (HCCA), which has grown in just a few years to more than 2,000 members and has taken steps to establish an academy and a certification process; (2) the Ethics Officers Association (EOA), which was founded in 1992 and has approximately 600 members; and, if you live in Australia, (3) the Association for Compliance Professionals of Australia (ACPA), which was founded in 1996 and currently has more than 300 members. Get involved and be one of the first to be certified, and help with mentoring new members.

Nimble networking also means maximizing your efforts in networking throughout your industry. Do industry recruiters and search professionals have you on file? Have you met them personally, and outlined your perfect job situation? Do you copy them or include them on your industry events and articles? Do you send them candidate leads and business when possible? Do you know the hiring executives, human resources professionals, and compliance colleagues at the companies that you have researched and targeted for your next career move? Invite them to a conference in which you are involved or ask them to participate in organizing an event. Send them updates on your industry's events. Find an opportunity to have an informational interview—perhaps a lunch to share ideas and career opportunities. Keep a current database, perhaps on your e-mail or a contact management system, where you can easily update your files and send something to them regularly. Do not forget holiday cards and thank you notes. As you get to know them better, send articles on their hobbies or outside interests.

Be a nimble networker in your community as well. A recent search conducted for an executive required the candidate to have exhibited a history in community service. Here is an assignment that you should really enjoy. Find an area of interest and a group with whom you want to become involved. If you cannot start at the board level, then start lower and work your way up. A good entry point in any charitable organization is to become involved with activities such as fund-raising, both because fund-raising is very needed and because this activity could give you reason to call your key contacts. You may also consider managing a charitable event internal to your organization, which will give you additional opportunities to network within your own company.

THE NIMBLE FINANCIAL FOUNDATION

Your financial stability is the foundation to your career and life plan. Nimble professionals have a solid financial foundation that allows them to make career and life choices free of financial pressure. Ideally, it frees you to quit a job when the timing is right without being concerned about the financial implications of such a move. If you believe your need for the financial security offered by your job is greater than the risk of leaving, the stress of staying may create job performance difficulties or tempt you to compromise ethical principles. Fear of loosing your job diminishes when you have a sound financial plan and the reserves to carry you through a new job search. Experts recommend that you have access to a minimum of six months' living expenses, in addition to your savings and retirement funds. How many professionals do you know who could afford to walk away from a job that compromised their integrity? The nimble professional could and would.

Again, whether you have a lot of money or a little, a plan is essential. Several professionals have retired before age 40 without an inheritance and without winning the lottery, while others with six-figure incomes struggle to make ends meet. When some moan about barely making it and how tough life is, books like Viktor Frankl's *Man's Search for Meaning, The Art of Happiness* by His Holiness the Dalai Lama and Howard C. Cutler, M.D., or *Simple Abundance* by Sarah Breathnach, can broaden their perspective so that they can more fully appreciate and enjoy their own situations. Even better, suggest that they help in a shelter for a few weeks. It does not hurt them to know that the median income of a family of four in the United States is less than $35,000 per year, and that out of the 30 fastest growing jobs categories in the booming economy, more than half of them pay less than $18,000 per year.[10] Many people do not understand how to put their money to work or even how money works at all. Some people have done very well learning to harness the power of money through groups like Debtor's Anonymous. This is a good way to become wise to your own spending habits and you do not need to be in debt to attend such a group and learn from their sound principles and methods.

Your first exercise for your financial freedom plan is to conduct an audit. Search the Internet and self-help books for help, and hire experts who will review your financial situation. Experts can teach sound financial principles, but be alert to their ulterior motives. One woman inherited $300,000, but knew nothing about money management or investing. Her financial auditor advised her to put her entire savings in a certificate of deposit, based on her age and lack of investment knowledge. Another client found out that he had confused money markets with mutual funds and was surprised to learn during his audit that his mutual funds were not insured. After your comprehensive audit, you may realize, like many of my clients, that you are not saving enough money. Finding the money to save is not always easy. You must live *below your means*.

Consider a recent national advertising campaign by SunAmerica, Inc., a leading retirement savings company. The advertising campaign takes aim at conspicuous consumption and taps into the human desire for immediate gratification by juxtaposing the costs of luxury goods with the potential value of the same amount of money put away for retirement or savings. In these ads, SunAmerica uses a hypothetical calculation on a $70,000 luxury car with an 8 percent pre-tax return compounded annually over 20 years. It is claimed that this $70,000 luxury car could be worth $326,000 in retirement savings. Another example is a beautiful luxury watch, costing $6,500. That watch could cost $30,000 in retirement or savings. SunAmerica conducted proprietary market research among 1,800 men and women that revealed that 61 percent of women and 53 percent of men said that they have little or no money to save for retirement after paying bills.[11] Yet many of these same people owned luxury cars, took expensive vacations, and spent a great deal on jewelry. People often do not know where their money goes. Remember the SunAmerica examples and start multiplying the cost of everything by five to decide whether you still *really* want it.

Retirement planning should be a critical part of your financial planning and considered in the foundation that you are creating. There are many factors to consider and discuss with your financial planner, including life expectancy, inflation, Social Security, your spending habits and plans, sources of income after retirement, and best- and worst-case scenarios. In your financial audit, calculate your probable needs at retirement and work backward to determine how and when you will get there. "How much is enough? A frugal retirement may fit you perfectly. Many middle class retirees do not need all their money. In other words, they have saved too much."[12]

> Look at what steps are between where you are now and where you want to be. Arrive at a realistic assessment of how much income you will need after retirement. Calculate how much you

are likely to receive from Social Security and other assured sources and a pension and then adopt a plan to close any retirement savings gap.[13]

THE NIMBLE IMAGE AND BEHAVIORAL PACKAGE

The author's interviews with top image and communication consultants and hiring executives have confirmed that an image package could be the single most powerful career advancement tool. Most experts say that an image package consists of physical appearance, professional behaviors, social graces, business etiquette, body language, and communication skills—the ability to speak, write, and listen well. Communicating effectively also means the timely delivery of and response to messages. The nimble professional seeks the complete package, continually striving for greater mastery in each area.

Your "Nimble Image Package" is a critical component of creating and enhancing your reputation and identity. You cannot take it too seriously. Participants in a second annual survey, titled "Profile of Health Care Compliance Officers," reported that 55 percent of compliance officers are at the senior management level, 17 percent are company officers, and 25 percent are in middle management.[14] It seems intuitively obvious that management representatives for their industries would be aware of how to dress, behave, and communicate appropriately with clients and others. However, this is not always the case. One of the reasons for the inconsistency is that compliance professionals come from many different backgrounds (that is, from teaching, health care administration, government, manufacturing, law, human resources, consulting, laboratory environments, and hospitals), some of which have a relatively casual dress style. Professionals from these fields may not be accustomed to an environment requiring executive attire and adherence to corporate protocol. The old saying, "Dress for the job you want," is true, as is its corollary, "Also dress and behave for the job you want to *keep!*"

A proper image or identity package is critical for professional success.[15] Every individual presents an image or identity of him- or herself that tells an immediate *story*, and that story carries a very strong message. Although each person's *personal story* is a combination of many things, such as behavioral characteristics (attitude, integrity, and dependability) and skill levels (relationship building, technical acumen, results-orientation, and work habits), the most evident and outward characteristics of who you are to the world is displayed through your visual, verbal, and nonverbal presentations.

Visual appearance includes the physical aspects of dress, style, and tone of voice, which in turn includes accent, vocabulary, pitch, speed, and volume. Verbal content refers to the actual words you choose to speak. What message is your package sending? How would others define your identity? Are all of the aspects of your package and presentation sending a *consistent* message?[16]

The moment you look at someone, you make initial judgments on appearances alone. Because initial contact with people is eye-to-body, everyone tends to evaluate clothes and body language first. Clearly then, because such profound value judgments are made from such superficial evidence, it would seem prudent to choose carefully the way you dress so that perceptions of you are favorable. Your personal and professional identity as a compliance professional needs to communicate credibility, trustworthiness, friendliness, and competence. Your professional presence needs to convey the whole message of your profession; namely, one of integrity and the pursuit of sound ethical and legal practices. You must "walk the talk" of your professional practice.[17]

A good common-sense appearance audit is to compare your *current look* with the *image of the time* by noticing the attire, hairstyles, and accessories of television news anchors, actors playing roles as executives, and role models in your own company and industry. Also notice how lean and fit they look. You might hire a fitness coach to measure your percentage of body fat, determine your fitness level, and give you feedback on posture and advice on nutrition, which will help maximize your health and energy levels. A coach can also create a program for you to manage stress and your overall image.

What about self-expression? Expressing yourself creatively is wonderful and usually best handled in the work environment through creatively and effectively excelling in your job. Think like the nimble professional, who sees the way you dress at work as an exquisite *uniform*—a uniform that expresses your quality, dependability, and the level of income that you want to earn. You may want to treat yourself to a few custom items for a tailored look, because off-the-rack clothing does not always fit perfectly. And fit is the key. Nothing sabotages an image worse than sleeves or pants that are too long or short. Get it all approved by an image consultant, if feasible, and see a good tailor for alterations. For creative expression, im-

age consultants and hiring executives in the compliance industry have recommended some freedom in ties for men, scarves and accessories for
women.

Behavior is also a part of your image package and career experts suggest
that the negative or problem behaviors listed below could devastate a career. Take the "Career Killers Audit." List each negative trait and describe
your actions to manage or neutralize *each* one:

- Look in the mirror—do you look healthy and fit? Did you get a fitness
  audit?
- What complaints, comments, or suggestions have associates, friends,
  and family made about your behavior? What will you do to enhance
  your behavior?
- Are you chronically late for meetings and with communications?
- Do you have poor communication procedures: you cannot be reached
  or do not return telephone calls or e-mails within 24 hours?
- Do you withhold information?
- Are you unable to make decisions within a reasonable time frame,
  letting opportunities pass?
- Are you withdrawing; have you hung up the telephone on someone or
  not been available?
- Do you have any addictions?
- Do you have credit problems? (Remember that many companies to-
  day do credit checks when hiring and promoting.)
- Do you violate procedures?
- Do you participate in illegal activities?
- Do you have a poor image? Did you do an image audit?
- Are you lying? (Never put false information on a job application or
  résumé; you will probably be found out and dismissed.)
- Do you gossip?
- Do you exhibit anger-based behavior or lose control of your temper?
- Do you miss deadlines?
- Do you blame others?

Now look back at the list of the attributes that describe the nimble professional listed in the first section. How do you measure up? Which ones
are missing? What will you do to enhance your behaviors?

The second important component in your image/identity package is
your nonverbal message, your body language and behaviors. As an exer-

cise, seek comments and coaching as part of an executive communications/presentation course. Such courses usually include your participation in a videotaped interview or presentation, with a subsequent critique. Also ask for feedback on body language from friends and family.

The third image/identity component is verbal content, which includes the command and selection of language. Today, many people do not have a good command of verbal and written communications. If you know this to be true about yourself, take some business writing courses and do vocabulary-building exercises. It may serve you well to verify your communications skills, asking for feedback from trusted professionals and seeking the advice of a professional writer or communications coach who will critique both your verbal and written communications. You may want to consider the composition techniques from the sales and marketing industry to teach yourself to sell your ideas more effectively. Check local universities and colleges for a professional writing coach, perhaps a professor or graduate student. Contact associations such as the International Association of Business Communicators and Women in Communications for referrals to communications experts and writers.[18] A professional writer or coach may assist you in enhancing résumés, cover letters, standard business correspondence, and the composition of articles. Use care in this process, however. Your approach to writing must be fully consistent with good ethical practice. Assistance in composing an article may help you improve your writing skills, but you could seriously damage your career if you take credit for someone else's writing that you publish under your own name.

THE NIMBLE INTERVIEW

Interviews are sales presentations on both the candidate's and the hiring company's sides. Both parties should view this as a great fact-finding, relationship, and public relations building opportunity, even when no offer is extended or accepted.

Face it. When you go to interviews, purchase decisions are being made. Employers see you and others to determine who they will acquire. Chances are an interviewer has at least read your résumé, which you or a recruiter sent. Now a salesperson is coming with the actual product. Get ready. They will not just look at the paint job and kick the tires. They will take a test drive! You are the salesperson. And you are also the product. Moreover, because it is an interview, not just a social call, your host has permission to probe deeply. They can ask tougher and more personal questions than they would ask at any other time. Your behavior and appearance will be scrutinized far more critically when you show up for an interview than on any ordinary work day in the next ten years.[19]

The company should make the candidate feel welcome and comfortable and give a brief but good sales presentation about the company, benefits, and career opportunities so that the candidate will leave with a good feeling about the company and take a positive message into the community. This is what *should* happen, but unfortunately due to ignorance and busy schedules it does not happen this way most of the time. However, do not let a poor interviewer spoil your presentation. Just keep it in your mind as a bad example and as a way not to handle interviews that you will conduct in the future.

Prepare for the interview as a salesperson would:

Just because you cannot deliver a salesperson's monologue is no reason not to prepare one. Analyze your product and your customer's needs, and develop the sales message you wish you could deliver in a 15-minute monologue. Then divide it into brief topical capsules. Almost every interviewer, no matter how inept, will ask questions that allow you to present everything you have in mind.[20]

Think like the company. Put yourself in the hiring person's mind, which will change as you move from the recruiter, to the human resources department, to the hiring department manager, to a corporate executive. Each interviewer will have specific needs and perceive certain risks associated with the hire. You must determine their needs and perceptions and talk into these areas to sell yourself, using your accomplishments, strengths, and skills.

You should have a clear idea of the job description or determine the company's needs early on in the interview, allowing you to augment your sales presentation with examples, case studies, and testimonials to show you are a potentially good hire. There are several types of interviews and most fall into one of two categories: (1) an informational or "kicking the tires" interview, and (2) the "real-thing," when you are applying for a definite opening. They are both sales presentations and should be handled similarly. Informational interviews are often mini-mentoring or career-counseling sessions where you meet to gain information on a company or industry or to discuss career opportunities, usually when there is no job opening advertised. This is a great way for candidates and companies to network and many hires do come from this type of a meeting. Although it is less formal, do not think for a minute that it is not an opportunity for you to position yourself into a job now or in the future. You may have an opportunity to ask something like, "What opportunities in compliance does your company offer and what are the requirements and responsibilities?" During the conversation—where you are doing a great deal of listening, just like any good salesperson—there will be opportunities for you to make your presentation.

Preparation is the key to all successful presentations, including interviews that are the "real thing." Create specific lists of pertinent questions that you will need to write answers to and rehearse, with a video camera if possible. Do not leave anything to chance. These questions will anticipate the objections you must overcome in your sales presentation/interview.

Also, do not put off learning how to present and sell yourself and your ideas until the week of an interview or presentation. Make sales excellence a part of your ongoing professional development, as you will need these skills in every aspect of your life. Prepare your "Evidence of Existence" information and your case studies. These are stories and summaries about projects or situations where you have demonstrated excellence. Give the project goals, details, your role, the solution(s) you or your team provided, and the end results. Weave these into your interview as examples and answers to questions. You might say, "Let me give you an example . . . ," and briefly tell your story or show your evidence.

If given an opportunity to ask questions, be prepared with a list of questions that show that you have researched the company, know the industry, and are qualified for this job. This may not be the right time to find out all the things that you want to know (for example, concerning benefits and "perks"), or it may be far enough along to ask when is the appropriate time to discuss or request information on those issues.

Salary negotiations can kill a good opportunity. Your goal is to get the best offer that you can, considering all criteria, not just money, while maintaining your dignity and the respect that you have earned. Often, making a lateral move or taking a pay cut can position you for a better long-term opportunity; however, this is usually not necessary. When a recruiter asks for your salary, tell them what you currently make, what you want to make, and sell them on why you are worth it. When a company requests salary information, it is appropriate to give them a range of current and expected salary and remind them that the salary is just a part of the package that you currently have and seek. Ask them, as part of your response, "What is the salary that they are considering for a *top performer?*" and say "That sounds appropriate," or "That matches what my research has shown," if this is true and the salary is in your range. This should keep discussions on the high end of the range. If the salary mentioned is too low, let the interviewer know what range you are seeking, but be aware that this may end the discussion.

You should also

> prepare a written summary of current compensation. It's as helpful as your résumé in orienting recruiters and employers. When do you hand over your compensation summary? Maybe never. The recruiter or the employer will surely ask, "What's your current compensation?" Answer with an approximate figure, justified by your summary. At that point the employer may say, "Well, that's in our ballpark. We can certainly come up with an attractive incentive." If so, don't go further. Pocket your summary and never pull it out. Obviously, you're going to get a tempting offer. On the other hand, your current compensation may spark a reaction like this: "Wow! That's certainly more than I would have thought. How do you come up with that number?"[21]

Use your summary at this point. If you are employed, your power in job and salary negotiations comes from your ability to indicate what a good deal you have in your current position. If you are not employed, using your most recent compensation package and industry research as part of your negotiating arsenal should bolster your confidence and credibility as long as your reason for being unemployed makes sense. If you have had to leave an employment situation on negative terms, try to negotiate a good reference if possible, or at least one that is neutral (that is, one where they verify only dates, job title, and basic information and state that this is company policy). You might consider sending a written request or having your attorney send a letter to the human resources department and your immediate past supervisor stating that you give permission to discuss only neutral information about your employment history, if you are in a negative situation. You may be able to get good letters of recommendation and good references from individuals in your company or industry professionals, and you should have your previous positive performance reviews and references from other jobs for your Interview Kit (discussed further below).

> Responsibility, growth opportunity, and possibly a chance to build long-term net worth, not just a boost in current income, will be your main reasons for any move. But you *do* expect financial improvement, both immediate and long-term. As an executive recruiter, I always make sure to find out every facet of current compensation, plus any expected changes within the next twelve months. And I communicate all of this information to my client company in a detailed written summary so that the client realizes, right from the start, that Candidate X will have to get upwards of $190,000 whereas Candidate Y can probably be hired for $130,000 and possibly less.[22]

In the interview, "bear in mind that you are proving yourself on two levels: as a fine person, and as someone obviously able to do the job."[23] Once an offer is extended, you can include special requests (for example, time off for your ski trip that is coming up in two months), if there has not been an opportunity to discuss these previously. In any case, all special requests should have been discussed earlier with your recruiter. You should request your offer in writing and get as much detail in writing as possible, as employment contracts are getting more difficult to negotiate. It can benefit you to accept the offer in writing, outlining your understanding of the position's requirements and the organization's offer and addressing areas that may have been overlooked in their letter. Senior executives should get an employment contract if possible,[24] approved by an attorney. Telephone screening and telephone interviews are becoming more prevalent. Prepare your family for the incoming call. Again, no kids, rude spouses, or roommates should answer the telephone, and you should prepare yourself with a quiet place to take the call where you can review and take notes. Have your résumé, case studies, salary/benefit breakdown report, and research on the company at your fingertips for these calls.

The time and day of the week can influence your interview's success. Try to schedule your interview Tuesdays through Thursdays, in the midmorning. Avoid late-afternoon meetings, which could conflict with your interviewer's schedule as his or her day comes to an end. Also, avoid hectic times such as the day before or after big holidays and heavy traffic times that could cause you to be late. Bring your "Interview Kit" to the interview, which includes additional copies of your résumé, an executive briefing (the high points of your résumé in a single narrative paragraph), letters of recommendation, your reference list, performance reviews, awards, copies of business presentations that you have made, reports and articles that you have written, and anything that is applicable to this particular job opportunity.[25] Do not hesitate to create a portfolio just as an architect might, with samples of work or photographs if applicable.

> Try to arrive ten minutes before your scheduled interview. If you arrive earlier, use your extra time to scope out the reception area resources. When the employer is late, be certain your appointment knows you have arrived. If half an hour goes by without the employer having materialized, and you must leave, take out a sheet of paper and write a polite note such as this: "Dear Mr. Smith: It is 10:35, and I assume that you have been unexpectedly and unavoidably detained. Perhaps we'd better reschedule our meeting. I'm at 000–000–0000. I'll check in with you later this afternoon." Sign the note, fold it in half, inscribe it clearly with Mr. Smith's name, and hand it to the receptionist. In a polite voice that betrays absolutely no trace of irritation, say, "Please be certain that Mr. Smith gets this note. We'll have to reschedule our appointment. Thanks very much." Keep this situation in perspective. You have every right to be angry if an employer is late for your interview, especially if he does not call to explain the situation. But anger will do you no good when the interviewer finally does show up. Forgive, forget, and get on with the interview.[26]

Finally, if possible, make an ally of the receptionist. The receptionist and the interviewers' assistants are important new friends, and they are often asked to deliver their opinion to the company's decision makers on how you handled yourself in the lobby or on the telephone. Realize that the interview actually starts as you drive into the parking lot. There are horror stories of anxious candidates giving an interviewer or prospective employer an angry word or inappropriate hand gesture while arguing over a parking spot. So relax. You are prepared, trained, and you have rehearsed. Your interviews and future presentations should go well.

THE NIMBLE PROFESSIONAL'S RÉSUMÉ PACKAGE

The nimble résumé package includes the résumé, cover letters, thank you letters, references, and choices of stationery. Consider these suggestions in preparing your résumé package. Avoid labels on envelopes as they look like junk mail. Use people's names and not their titles. Make sure that the names are spelled correctly. Fax and e-mail your résumé to several associates to confirm its clarity before actually using it. Use large, clear fonts, especially for your name and telephone numbers. Bring several résumés to the interview. You can consider using any one of five formats for the résumé: (1) chronological, (2) functional, (3) achievement, (4) hybrid based on the chronological format, or (5) hybrid based on the functional format. See *The Complete Idiot's Guide to the Perfect Resume* for more details on types of résumés.[27] The most important section of your résumé is the first section—the Executive Summary for a seasoned professional or the Highlights section for a new graduate. This section should bullet point your achievements and special skills. You could put your Education section under the Summary of Qualifications section near the beginning of the résumé if your education is highly relevant to the new position. (See Appendix 12–A for an example of a well-written résumé.)

Cover Letters. Senior Vice President Charles Nagle of Tyler & Company, a national executive search firm specializing in health care, often uses the cover letter as part of the screening process.[28] Remember that your written and verbal skills will be assessed at every turn of the interview process, so verify and enhance your skills whenever possible. If you hire a typist or even a résumé/cover letter service, request a diskette with copies of your work, written in software compatible with most current computers. The cost should be only a few dollars. Get a signed letter of agreement with the service at the beginning of the process to set the price, the scope of the project, delivery times and procedures, and retention period for records. Negotiate a discount if they run late in delivery, which often happens in smaller résumé writing companies and with individuals who write or type as a part-time job.

Follow-up or "Re-Sell" Letters. This letter is basically a thank you for the interview, but it is also an opportunity to "re-sell" yourself. Make sure to include specifics on how your background matches the job description. Remind the interviewer of any areas where you both agreed there was a match. Thank them for the opportunity and information that you received and state how you look forward to moving to the next step. Choose something a little heavier than 20 pound paper, but not as thick as card stock.[29] Grey or cream colored paper are acceptable choices.

Networking Résumé Cards. "A networking card is a hybrid between a résumé and a business card. It is an ideal marketing tool when a résumé is too long and a business card does not say enough."[30] For the unemployed, these serve as a business card. A good printing company or copy store can easily and inexpensively print these on a color copier and cut them into business size or slightly larger cards with your contact information on the front and highlights of your résumé on the back. These cards are great for networking meetings and it is a good idea to send one with your résumé and regular business card. Do not use home-printed cards with perforated edges.

More Tidbits. "Commandment V: 'Thou shalt not lie.' Getting caught with your hand in the cookie jar could put your job on the line."[31] "You can embellish within certain limits, but do not lie in your interview or on your résumé. Avoid using the phrase 'responsible for.' This phrase does not clearly describe your level of involvement. Did you think of an idea that others carried out, or did you work overtime to implement every detail of a project? Be sure to give yourself full credit by using action verbs to indicate exactly what your role was."[32]

Now that you know about the nimble professional, you have more insight into why some people get ahead while others, often those who are more qualified and work just as hard, are left behind. Take the suggestions and give them a try. See what fits for you. Get some consultants and coaches to help. Follow your head and heart, and create a wonderful career and life.

NOTES

1. This is also the current working title of a book in progress by the author.
2. Webster's Encyclopedia Unabridged Dictionary of the English Language at 1300 (1996).
3. J. Lucht, The New Rites of Passage at $100,000+: The Insiders Lifetime Guide to Executive Job-Changing and Faster Career Progress at 347 (1999).

4. S.R. COVEY, PRINCIPLE-CENTERED LEADERSHIP 33–38 (1990).

5. S.R. COVEY, PRINCIPLE-CENTERED LEADERSHIP 42 (1990).

6. J.D. POND, THE NEW CENTURY FAMILY MONEY BOOK: YOUR COMPREHENSIVE GUIDE TO A LIFETIME OF FINANCIAL SECURITY 247 (1993).

7. J.D. POND, THE NEW CENTURY FAMILY MONEY BOOK: YOUR COMPREHENSIVE GUIDE TO A LIFETIME OF FINANCIAL SECURITY 254 (1993).

8. J.D. POND, THE NEW CENTURY FAMILY MONEY BOOK: YOUR COMPREHENSIVE GUIDE TO A LIFETIME OF FINANCIAL SECURITY 254 (1993).

9. S.R. COVEY, PRINCIPLE-CENTERED LEADERSHIP 102–104 (1990).

10. J. HIGHTOWER, IF THE GODS HAD MEANT US TO VOTE THEY WOULD HAVE GIVEN US CANDIDATES 152 (2000).

11. Available on the Internet at <http://www.sunamerica.com>.

12. R. WARNER, GET A LIFE: YOU DO NOT NEED A MILLION TO RETIRE 3 (1996).

13. R. WARNER, GET A LIFE: YOU DO NOT NEED A MILLION TO RETIRE 159 (1996).

14. TYLER & COMPANY AND WALKER INFORMATION, PROFILE OF HEALTH CARE COMPLIANCE OFFICERS 11 (1999).

15. Susan McLeay and Lynne Henderson, partners with the author in CEO International, Inc., Atlanta, Georgia.

16. The author thanks Susan McLeay, partner in CEO International, Inc., for these observations.

17. The author thanks Lynne Henderson, image and communications expert, past president of Association of Image Consultants International (AICI), owner of the London Image Institute, and partner in CEO International, Inc., for these observations. See also J. LUCHT, THE NEW RITES OF PASSAGE AT $100,000+: THE INSIDERS LIFETIME GUIDE TO EXECUTIVE JOB-CHANGING AND FASTER CAREER PROGRESS 302 (1999).

18. Available on the Internet at <http://www.iabc.com and http://www.wic.com>.

19. J. LUCHT, THE NEW RITES OF PASSAGE AT $100,000+: THE INSIDERS LIFETIME GUIDE TO EXECUTIVE JOB-CHANGING AND FASTER CAREER PROGRESS 345–46 (1999).

20. J. LUCHT, THE NEW RITES OF PASSAGE AT $100,000+: THE INSIDERS LIFETIME GUIDE TO EXECUTIVE JOB-CHANGING AND FASTER CAREER PROGRESS 351 (1999).

21. J. LUCHT, THE NEW RITES OF PASSAGE AT $100,000+: THE INSIDERS LIFETIME GUIDE TO EXECUTIVE JOB-CHANGING AND FASTER CAREER PROGRESS 378–80 (1999).

22. J. LUCHT, THE NEW RITES OF PASSAGE AT $100,000+: THE INSIDERS LIFETIME GUIDE TO EXECUTIVE JOB-CHANGING AND FASTER CAREER PROGRESS 378–80 (1999).

23. J. LUCHT, THE NEW RITES OF PASSAGE AT $100,000+: THE INSIDERS LIFETIME GUIDE TO EXECUTIVE JOB-CHANGING AND FASTER CAREER PROGRESS 346 (1999).

24. See Chapter 8, Protecting Yourself and Your Profession.

25. M. DORIO, THE COMPLETE IDIOT'S GUIDE TO THE PERFECT INTERVIEW 35–36 (1997).

26. M. DORIO, THE COMPLETE IDIOT'S GUIDE TO THE PERFECT INTERVIEW 58–58 (1997).

27. S. IRELAND, THE COMPLETE IDIOT'S GUIDE TO THE PERFECT RESUME 227 (1996).

28. Tyler & Company, Atlanta, Georgia; available on the Internet at <http://www.tylerandco.com>.

29. S. IRELAND, THE COMPLETE IDIOT'S GUIDE TO THE PERFECT RESUME 185 (1996).

30. S. IRELAND, THE COMPLETE IDIOT'S GUIDE TO THE PERFECT RESUME 40–41 (1996).

31. S. IRELAND, THE COMPLETE IDIOT'S GUIDE TO THE PERFECT RESUME 159 (1996).

32. S. IRELAND, THE COMPLETE IDIOT'S GUIDE TO THE PERFECT RESUME 135 (1996).

Sample Hybrid Chronological Achievement, Functional Résumé

John Sample
233 Apple Drive
Mableton, Georgia 30188
Home # (770) 000-0000
Work # (770) 000-0000 ext. 203
E-mail: Jsample@boohoo.com

Objective: Health Care Chief Compliance Officer position.

EXECUTIVE SUMMARY

Senior health care professional with record of progress, promotion, and achievement in health care finance, reimbursement, auditing, consulting, and information systems. Corporate officer responsible for compliance with laws, regulations, and policies for Medicare (Part A & Part B) and Medicaid programs in two public companies with combined revenues of $6 billion from a full spectrum of services including acute care, home health pharmacy, and other specialty services. More than 8 years' experience with accomplishments with Medicare Intermediary.

Major experience, strengths, and skills include:

- Developed and implemented an MIS System, Accounting consolidation system that cut costs by + $1 M in 1999 and increased revenue collection $3 M in the 1st and 2nd quarter 2000.

Courtesy of Tyler & Company, Atlanta, Georgia.

253

- Developed and implemented strategies that increased profits by more than $2 M.
- Designed new marketing and sales materials that increased sales by $5 M in 1999.
- Directed the development of the first DRG system in the industry.
- Reduced department turnover from 32% per quarter in 1998 to 10% per quarter in 1999 and 5% in 2000.
- Directed merger with $10 M health care system
- Keynote speaker at HCCA International conference.

EXPERIENCE

ABC Company   1993–2000

ABC Company is a fast-growing public company that provides skilled nursing care and specialty medical services, including rehabilitation, sub-acute care, home health, long term acute care, pharmacy, wound care, and IV therapies.

Senior Vice President—Chief Information Officer (CIO)

Reported to President & Chairman

Responsible for developing and implementing information systems and technology strategies for an integrated health care information system designed to support the strategic objectives and to provide access to management, financial, and clinical information across the enterprise. Accomplishments included:

- Developed and implemented Company's information systems and technology plan, which focused on the need to gather more financial, operational, and clinical information quicker and more accurately to achieve a competitive edge in the rapidly changing health care environment.
- Consolidated facility patient accounting/AR systems.
- Implemented systems for management key indicator reporting, labor trend and analysis, financial forecasting, e-mail, and clinical reporting.

Vice President—Director of Reimbursement & Information Systems

Reported to President

Corporate officer responsible for compliance with laws, regulations, and policies of the federal Medicare and state Medicaid programs. Responsible for developing, recommending, and implementing business strategies and plans for optimizing reimbursement, profitability, and productivity under Medicaid, Medicare, managed care, and other third-party payer programs. Approved company's managed care contracts. Directed the ABC Hospital's MIS department to provide quality management, financial, and clinical information systems technology to support the goals and objectives. Accomplishments included:

- Reorganized the reimbursement department and in three months achieved the highest satisfaction ratings ever received by the department.
- Directed the implementation of strategies and plans, which increased profits by more than $2 M (documented), and substantially increased cash flow.
- Played key role in improving the payer mix and profitability. Maximized Medicare reimbursement for increased higher level of medical services.
- Directed the successful filing of more than $1.5 M in RCL exceptions.

XYZ Consulting   1992–1993

Consultant

XYZ Consulting provided consulting and information services to the health care industry. The Company specialized in managed care and its services and products included: management consulting, mergers & acquisitions, strategic planning, industry and company reports, and seminars. Served as independent consultant to Company. Accomplishments included:

- Performed strategic planning and acquisition reviews for hospital clients seeking to purchase health maintenance organizations (HMOs).

Identified and analyzed potential acquisition candidates, completed valuation and pricing assessments, developed negotiation and acquisition strategy recommendations, recommended structuring, developed due diligence plans, and performed due diligence.
- Designed new marketing and sales materials for company's information services and products.

Sample Inc.   1977–1985

Corporate Vice President—Director Information Systems Planning

Reported to CFO

Responsible for the development of the Company's information systems architecture and the management strategies and plans necessary for its implementation. Had the responsibility to ensure that the Company's information systems resources were aligned with the corporate strategic goals and objectives, and that expected system benefits were achieved. Accomplishments included:

- Created and chaired information systems steering committee composed of senior managers representing all areas of Company operations. Developed the company's first information systems strategic plan.
- Directed development of one of the first DRG optimization systems in the industry.
- Directed development or modification of a wide variety of systems: financial reporting, patient care information, integrated purchasing and payments, cost accounting, A/R collections, dietary, et al.
- Organized and managed business systems planning group, which consulted with users on systems needs and made recommendations on new systems or modification of existing systems.

Sample Inc.   1974–1977

Assistant Director—Reimbursement

Reported to Vice President of MIS

Responsible for managing staff, which interpreted and determined applicability of laws, regulations, and pronouncements, handled Medicare litigation and appeals, and reviewed procedures of audit staff to ensure compliance with laws and regulations. Accomplishments included:

- Negotiated settlement of more than $5 M in disputes with Medicare providers.
- Planned, organized, and conducted training programs and seminars for health care providers, physicians, and in-house staff.

Sample Inc. 1970–1973

Manager, Plan Settlement and Reimbursement

Responsible for managing staff, which resolved complex accounting and reimbursement problems, developed comments on proposed law and regulations, provided consulting and training, conducted performance audits, handled litigation and appeals, reviewed and negotiated budgets, and reviewed and approved audit subcontracts. One of two individuals responsible for organizing a Medicare operation to replace the one being operated by Sample Inc. Accomplishments included contracting for office space and equipment, hiring and training personnel, subcontracting audits, determining final settlement amounts for Medicare providers, establishing claims processing system, and provider relations and consulting.

EDUCATION

MBA, College or University
B.S. Finance, College or University

MEMBERSHIPS

Health Care Compliance Association
Healthcare Information and Management Systems Society
Healthcare Financial Management Association

Community Service:[1]

Hobbies and Interests:[1]

---

[1]These sections are optional. Include only if relevant to the job at hand or if it shows particular leadership or athletic achievement.

CHAPTER 13

So You Want To Work in the Health Care Compliance Field: Practical Advice on Developing a Career in Health Care Compliance

Anne Adams

Every so often exciting opportunities emerge to participate in the development of new areas in an industry. It helps to be aware of upcoming trends, but, for the health care industry, the careers in the compliance arena seemed to have emerged over night. Other industries have compliance officers—brokerage firms and the environmental and defense industries—so compliance departments and programs are not new.

With the advent of corporate integrity agreements, and with the development of compliance guidances by the Department of Health and Human Services (HHS) Office of Inspector General (OIG) for all areas of the health care industry, a high-level compliance official charged with overseeing compliance has become a necessary component of any health care organization's executive leadership team. Perhaps other people in the organization already have been involved in the elements of a compliance program, such as training and educating, or auditing and monitoring.

Jobs in the compliance arena of the health care industry continue to provide new career opportunities. Although some providers had compliance programs in place in the early 1990s, they were usually government mandated. Not until the move for the development and implementation of voluntary health care compliance programs did the field begin to offer career opportunities for a variety of people with varying backgrounds as great as the variety of their skill sets. Backgrounds of compliance industry professionals may include law, accounting, finance, education, clinical (nurses and physicians), risk management, and quality assurance, to name just a few.

Academic medical centers, hospitals, home health agencies, nursing homes, physician practices, and third-party billing companies, as well as others in the health care industry, have developed and are still continuing to develop voluntary compliance programs. This continued effort will increase the demand for various types of professional compliance staff to work in these organizations, and for professional advice from outside the organization.

Also, the government and private sector side of the equation should not be overlooked. As the initiative on the fight against health care fraud and abuse continues, there will be an increased need in the government and private sector for investigators and enforcers. There are career opportunities with the Federal Bureau of Investigation (FBI), OIG, Department of Justice, and various state agencies. Opportunities with government contractors, such as the Medicare carriers and intermediaries, are also available, as well as with private commercial payers.

ASSESSING PERSONAL COMPATIBILITY WITH THE HEALTH CARE COMPLIANCE FIELD

Many individuals currently working in the health care field find compliance interesting and challenging, and a welcome change of pace compared with the traditional health care areas in which they have worked. An individual who is contemplating entering the compliance field should do several things to assess personal compatibility with the compliance profession.

First, someone considering work in the compliance field should ask him- or herself, "Why do I want to be in this field?" Whether currently in health care or thinking of switching careers, this is a question that must be answered. Make a list of the pros and cons of changing careers or changing jobs within health care. Talk to those who are already in the compliance field. It may take some time and commitment to learn the "compliance ropes" if a person has not worked in the health care field before, or if an individual has not been in a part of health care organization that has been heavily investigated by the government, but it can be done.

Each individual also will need to assess the type of personality that he or she has. In addition, the personality of the potential employing health care organization must be assessed. Investigate what type of program it wants to develop or what type of program it already has in place. Try to assess the type of person and personality the organization wants to run the program.

Does the organization want a compliance department that can facilitate change and train and educate staff, or does it want a compliance enforcement department? This truly is an important question to consider, because if the compliance officer's philosophy of compliance differs from the organization's philosophy, then it will not be a good fit.

Also, consider these questions: Do I have thick skin? Can I accept criticism? Can I make decisions that may be unpopular and meet with resistance? Am I a detail-oriented person? Can I gain the trust of people and build consensus? Can I delegate, manage multiple projects at the same time, analyze problems, and create effective solutions to address them? Can I speak in front of groups and teach adult learners? And, most important, am I willing to roll up my sleeves and get in the trenches to make things happen? If the answer to these questions is "yes," then a career in the health care compliance field may be a good choice!

TYPES OF JOBS IN THE HEALTH CARE COMPLIANCE FIELD

The most recognizable position in the compliance profession is that of the chief compliance officer (CCO). The CCO usually oversees the organization's compliance department. In addition to the CCO, a compliance department may have an associate compliance officer, an assistant director of compliance, a compliance coordinator, a compliance trainer, a compliance manager, and/or compliance auditors who are skilled in physician and hospital coding and billing requirements. Positions within the department vary from organization to organization.

Organizations may look for employees with certain types of professional backgrounds, depending on the role to be filled in the organization's compliance department. Compliance departments may consist of attorneys, accountants, former government employees, nurses, and/or hospital administrators. An advanced degree in health care administration and practical health care operations experience is an advantage in health care compliance. A person with that type of background is able to understand the dynamics in which an organizational compliance program operates. A background in operations provides practical, real life-experience, which in turn provides insight in designing processes and developing workable compliance programs.

For example, an organization may want to enlist the assistance of a laboratory manager to work on the laboratory compliance team. He or she may be the ideal candidate to be the laboratory compliance program manager because of his or her knowledge of day-to-day laboratory operations and can best integrate compliance into the overall system; it may become part of the job with some type of reporting responsibility to the compliance department.

The compliance industry also has opportunities for consultants, but a consultant must be willing to travel—usually five days per week. A consultant may also be expected to help sell the products of the consulting firm. Some consultants leave consulting for an in-house position with a compliance department, but for many who take that route there is a decrease in pay and so they eventually leave the organization and return to consulting.

The industry indications are that many health care providers have already filled their CCO positions. Of course, these types of positions are still available or will become available as compliance officers leave to take other positions or enter other fields. Again, many compliance officers may leave the industry to join consulting firms; others leave to join law firms or accounting firms.

However, many professionals searching for a position as a compliance officer find that they cannot get the CCO position. So where should they look to be a part of this growing and exciting field? One area to consider is training, which is a component of many compliance departments. Depending on an organization's size, there may be a need for full-time compliance training. Not only is this a possibility internally within a health care organization, but it is also possible—depending on an individual's skills—to contract with other facilities that need training but do not necessarily need a full-time trainer.

Another training area is the development of training materials. Many companies are now developing education software for a variety of areas and health care compliance is certainly a field that is ready for such applications. Software development of compliance resources for use on the Internet is a rapidly developing area. Compliance software development or course writing may be a career opportunity for a person who has technical skills and a health care background.

The publication of the OIG Small Group Practice Guidance[1] will also lead to new opportunities, as well. Small group practices may need assistance in conducting risk assessments, auditing, and developing a compliance program that is right for them. Small group practices usually do not have large consulting budgets and would be unable to retain some of the larger consulting companies, so there is an opportunity for smaller consulting companies as well as for individuals to obtain independent contractor jobs.

In an interview with the author, Mary Wynkoop, Senior Vice President with Meridian Executive Search, confirms that people looking for positions in compliance often cannot get the CCO job. She surmises that most organizations have those positions filled, and suggests that those interested in compliance look to the field of e-commerce security. This area is rising to the top of many organizations' compliance focus. She reports that organizations are focusing on security issues both in the financial and patient information areas. She also suggests that people looking for positions explore opportunities in the corporate world, such as in the pharmaceutical industry, in medical equipment manufacturing companies, or in health care software companies. The Health Insurance Portability and Accountability Act's (HIPAA)[2] security and privacy requirements are probably driving this focus. In fact, the proposed privacy regulations require that an organization appoint a privacy officer.

Another job that is emerging as a new career opportunity in the compliance field is the coding and financial specialist. Whether it is physician or hospital billing, or cost report or chargemaster review, having these specialized skills are much sought after by health care organizations. Susan Minchew, CPC (Certified Professional Coder), Assistant Director of Billing Compliance for Emory Healthcare, recommends that people interested in a career in coding obtain certification. She also suggests that a coder should expand his or her knowledge base to include hospital coding and teaching physician guidelines in order to be more valuable to an employer.

Gina Seewald, with Meridian Staffing, places people with coding skills in temporary to permanent positions and agrees with Ms. Minchew. She indicates that there is a shortage of professional coders in the industry. Traditionally, coders have been mostly women, and there is a current trend under way for coders to work from home. According to Ms. Seewald, software development, electronic medical records, and the Internet will permit such work arrangements.

Health information management is another growing field within the health care compliance arena. With continued changes in reimbursement, continued development of electronic medical record information, and the privacy and security laws, health information specialists will be much sought after in the health care industry. A four-year degree in this area is available. Someone who is just starting a college program, contemplating earning a degree for the first time, or thinking about earning an additional degree might explore the field of health information management.

Someone who enjoys working behind the scenes should explore the possibility of writing articles for trade journals, including medical, legal, and compliance reports. Such an individual must have or develop good interviewing and writing skills, be willing to go after a story, and be accurate and able to meet deadlines. Check with the various publishing houses to see what they have available and send in a writing sample that is relevant to the publication.

RESOURCES

Each state should have a hospital or health system association that should be able to provide a list of all the hospitals and health systems in that state. Many associations also have regulatory attorneys or coordinators who are "in tune" with state and federal issues, including compliance. These associations should be able to provide some literature and lists of health care providers. Also, some hospitals and all academic medical centers have libraries that may have such information; the librarians are usually very helpful. Also, remember to investigate physicians' professional associations.

Membership in organizations that have a compliance theme also keeps the potential compliance professional in touch with the industry's trends and needs. Consider joining the Health Care Compliance Association, the American Health Lawyers Association, Health Financial Management Association, or the American Association of Professional Coders, and be sure to check out the local and affiliate associations, too. Attend meetings and talk to people in these organizations. Be willing to participate on committees and offer to participate in conferences or be a member of the conference development team.

The following helpful "Top 14 Tips" for finding a position within the health care compliance field are the result of life experience and numerous interviews:

1. Talk with people who are already in the health care field about working in the compliance area and seek their opinions and guidance. Most people are willing to meet with someone who is re-

searching the opportunity to enter a new field. However, never turn these meetings into job interviews.

2. Read all the OIG Guidances—they provide a lot of background information as well as knowledge about industry-specific compliance issues. This will provide a general base of knowledge for discussion with potential employers.

3. Read the major laws that govern health care compliance issues.

4. Read the relevant trade journals to keep up-to-date on what is happening in the industry and to keep abreast of advertised career opportunities. Such journals are available at the libraries of universities that have any type of clinical or administrative health care program.

5. Attend a health care compliance seminar, whether national or local. If time and money are limiting factors, there are many very good local seminars. Local law firms will also sometimes offer compliance seminars, as well as local chapters of national professional organizations. Many of the large law firms have Web sites that advertise upcoming conferences, which are often free of charge.

6. Invest in a membership in one or more of the compliance associations.

7. "Surf" the Internet. There is a lot of information on the Internet, including compliance information and job postings.

8. Join health care compliance list servers. They provide information on hot topics in the health care compliance arena and connect people electronically with whom to network.

9. Explore employment opportunities with placement or recruiting firms. These firms may have been retained to fill specific positions.

10. Look into the increasing opportunities in the government sector, especially for those with financial, legal, or other needed skills. With all the corporate integrity agreements in place, the government may have needs for enforcement staff.

11. Seek out those organizations that have government-imposed compliance programs. The list can be found on the OIG Web page, http://www.os.dhhs.gov/progorg/oig/cia/ciaoct.htm. Take a look at the corporate integrity agreements and the requirements of the agreements. Such organizations may need individuals with certain skill sets.

12. When approaching an organization, go with a presentation of personal skills, strengths, and ideas.

13. Become a specialist in a particular compliance area; for example, become a HIPAA security or privacy expert.
14. Create a compliance position! If already employed by an organization (not just in health care) that should develop and implement a compliance program, do the research, develop a proposal, create a budget, and present the recommendation to management.

NOTES

1. Department of Health and Human Services, Office of Inspector General, Compliance Program Guidance for Individual and Small Group Physician Practices (Sept. 2000), <http://www.hhs.gov/oig/modcomp/index.htm>.
2. 42 U.S.C. § 1320d-2; 45 C.F.R. Parts 160–164.

CHAPTER 14

Managing Organizational and Individual Conduct: The Politics of Compliance

Randal J. Dennings

> Man is by nature a political animal.
>
> Aristotle

INTRODUCTION

Compliance is traditionally described or perceived as a management discipline whose object is, among other things, to manage both organizational and individual conduct. However, there is a further dimension of compliance that is not traditionally articulated, namely, the compliance professional's skillful use of "applied psychology" as a *political strategy* to achieve desired outcomes when managing both organizational and individual conduct. This chapter addresses some aspects of the "politics of compliance" that are inherent in every compliance professional's job.

I address the politics of compliance from a practical or experiential perspective rather than an academic or theoretical perspective. A practicing lawyer for more than 20 years, I have been privileged to be part of and to advise compliance and audit committees and compliance professionals for more than 15 of those years. In this regard, particularly on the basis of my participation on compliance committees, I consider myself part of the emerging compliance profession. Accordingly, my comments here have been forged in the crucible of practical experience where clients quickly discarded an idea if it did not provide immediately perceived "added value." In a recent lecture on compliance to a class in the Master of Laws program at the University of New South Wales,[1] I described my approach as essentially one of a "mature lifeguard," providing practical tips to a class of "potential lifeguards." By taking this practical approach, I hope that the reader will be spared some of the pitfalls out of which the author has had painfully to scramble!

That said, I will argue here that there appears to be a "blurring" of organizational and individual goals, objectives, and conduct in compliance.[2] This means that there appears to be a dichotomy between the real goals and objectives of organizations and individuals and their actual conduct. Compliance professionals should learn to recognize this dichotomy and to harness it for the benefit of their organization and its particular compliance culture. It may well be that by doing so the relevant individual within the organization may also benefit. In any case, the political methods by which compliance professionals approach their tasks will vary with their organizations' cultures and the skills and attributes of each individual compliance professional. The first part of this chapter examines this briefly. The second part of the chapter develops these themes and draws upon four case studies of actual compliance professionals to illustrate some of the practical implications of compliance politics.

THE BLURRING BETWEEN GOALS AND OBJECTIVES VERSUS CONDUCT: THE "GOALS V. CONDUCT MATRIX"

As illustrated in Figure 14–1, from both an organizational and individual perspective there regularly appears a "blurring" between articulated goals and objectives and actual conduct.

When working closely with an organization, it is initially quite easy to determine the publicly articulated goals and objectives of the organization. These reside in mission statements, annual reports, and staff and customer publications. However, after working with an organization for some time, it often becomes apparent that there are at least two further sets of goals and objectives. First, there are the goals and objectives that are only privately articulated within the organization. Second, in some instances there are *real but hidden* organizational goals and objectives that are usually not publicly articulated and sometimes not even privately articulated.

In many instances, an organization's privately articulated goals and objectives may simply be those goals and objectives that are promulgated by separate sections or business units of the organization. An example of a privately articulated objective is a business development section's plan to discourage a particular category of customer in favor of another category

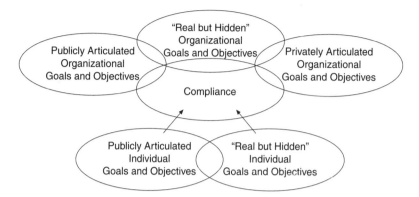

Figure 14–1 The Blurring of Articulated Goals and Objectives and Actual Conduct.

of customer. Although such a plan might improve the overall organization's profitability, it also might not be appropriate to publicize. In Australia, for instance, certain national financial institutions use such strategies to maximize the development of close customer relationships with high net worth individuals and to discourage the development of rural customers. Although no doubt a profitable move, these strategies could be damaging from a publicity perspective if they became known.

An example of the "real but hidden" organizational goals and objectives that are neither publicly nor even privately articulated within major parts of the organization can be seen in many organizations' unspoken, but nevertheless genuine, long-term objectives to replace expensive labor costs (and therefore employees) by using more technology and outsourcing. Because of the sensitive nature of this strategy, its existence is often kept a closely guarded secret from all but the inner circles of the organization's leadership. It is hidden, but real.

Sometimes there is also a dichotomy between the publicly articulated and the "real but hidden" *individual* goals and objectives of persons, both manager and nonmanager alike, working within organizations. In essence, some people do not fully and truthfully articulate their real goals and objectives. The reasons for this are many, including the following:

- the failure by some individuals to develop fully and adopt *any* clearly articulated goals and objectives for their lives or careers

- the personality characteristics of the individuals are such that, either from shyness or malevolence, they cannot publicly articulate their privately held goals and objectives
- the corporate culture of the organization renders such declarations inappropriate or, indeed, quite counterproductive (this could be because either these statements are thought to be naïve or are simply "not the way we do things around here")

Thus, there appears to be a potentially volatile matrix of conflicting goals and objectives at play in organizations about which compliance professionals need not only to be aware, but also need to master. They master such conflicts, in part, by the development and application of political skills. In this way, they can successfully achieve their own and their employing organization's compliance objectives. Thus, one of the major roles for compliance professionals is to identify and deal with the "blurring" of the public, private, and "real but hidden" goals and objectives as they relate to organizational and individual conduct.

Many organizations put excellent compliance programs in place that successfully embed compliance principles into operational procedures. The difficulty occurs on the behavioral level where, for a whole host of reasons—not the least of which is the blurring described earlier—individuals simply do not comply with the articulated operational procedures.[3] A healthy compliance culture can sharpen the focus of the organizational goals and objectives and thereby reduce the amount of blurring. And this, in turn, can build on itself, removing the organization's motives for hiding its goals and objectives. In any case, healthy compliance cultures tend to promote the "truthful" or focused articulation of organizational goals and objectives that, in turn, tends at the same time to foster a culture that not only welcomes and encourages individuals to promote their own goals and objectives, but also seeks to harness them for organizational purposes.

Indeed, much of the employee cynicism directed toward a compliance program's goals and objectives within an organization might actually be a byproduct of employee disillusionment from having been "burnt" previously. This can occur when employees trust the organization's publicly articulated goals and objectives and worked consistently with them, only to find that they were not the real goals and objectives of the organization and thus that their behavior in support of the articulated goals and objectives was therefore not appropriate and that they suffered for it. The successful compliance professional will learn to operate within this matrix of organizational and individual cross-currents.

A question remains, however, for the compliance professional to consider. If an organization has a significant "blurring" of public, private, and "real but hidden" goals and objectives in the sense described earlier, can it in fact have a healthy compliance culture? If, as contended earlier, a high degree of blurring is indicative of a *poor* compliance culture, then it may be that no matter how skillful the compliance professional, a successful compliance program may be next to impossible to achieve. In fact, an organization with a poor compliance culture or that has leaders who lack the organizational will to improve that culture dramatically and quickly will render even the most determined compliance "super champion" impotent. Without "commitment from the top" the compliance program will almost certainly fail. It will fail because short-term compliance concerns will always overrule long-term compliance concerns in this type of culture. Ultimately, this will cause compliance professionals to lose heart, self-respect, and perhaps even their reputations. As one compliance professional stated, "Life's too short to work in a habitually noncompliant organization."

Essentially, then, each organization's culture, whether public or private, will dictate the compliance professional's appropriate style of politicking. Thus, it might be said that each organization "gets the compliance culture that it deserves." If this is true, then each organization's culture tends to dictate, select, or develop the compliance candidate who exhibits its own style. The healthier the culture of an organization, the more clearly focused are both its organizational and individual goals and objectives. This means that "real" organizational goals and objectives are more likely to be publicly and privately articulated and not "hidden."[4] From an individual perspective there is no organizational need to dissimulate individual goals and objectives. Interestingly, a healthy organizational culture often leads to higher formal status and "clout" for the compliance professional, although, particularly in smaller organizations, the compliance professional can still have significant status and "clout" through the expert use of informal methods of internal politicking.

SOME SUCCESSFUL MANAGEMENT EXAMPLES OF COMPLIANCE POLITICKING

Granted the dynamic organizational and individual matrix described earlier, how do successful compliance professionals creatively and constructively use politics to further their own and their organizations' compliance objectives? There is no "one-size-fits-all" answer or approach. Each organization presents an appropriate solution given its compliance and organizational cultures, and the personal characteristics of its successful compliance professional. This chapter will continue to use the practical approach by examining four real compliance professionals. These professionals have some or all of the Australian Standards' list of ideal attributes.[5] To ensure anonymity, these four compliance professionals will be identified by the following descriptions: The Corporate Leader ("A"); The Blue Collar Leader ("B"); The Quiet Achiever ("C"); and The Traffic Cop ("D").

It should be stressed at this point that all these compliance professionals were and are extremely successful, if success is defined as not only achieving a high rate of operational compliance within the organization, but also achieving this result in a manner that increased the health of the compliance culture generally and addressed other important organizational objectives as well. For example, one compliance professional implemented a new compliance process in such a way as to not only achieve the desired compliance outcome, but also did so in conjunction with training for another purpose, thereby significantly minimizing costs. Another re-engineered some of the organization's operational procedures so as to make them far simpler for staff and customers to use while implementing the compliance program. This, in turn, increased the organization's market share and customer satisfaction, while also improving employee productivity. In any case, the four compliance professionals may be described as follows.

The Corporate Leader. "A" was the perfect corporate senior management woman, recently employed by the company for a senior position, although not in compliance. She presented efficiently and effectively, and has an MBA degree and business background. Compliance was a problem with the company as it had grown quickly and desperately needed to put operational procedures in place to ensure compliance. "A" was asked to do the job by the chief executive officer (CEO) of the organization even though she had no previous experience in compliance.

With her usual enthusiasm, "A" quickly reviewed the available literature and drew up a detailed project plan. "A" then sought expert compliance consulting services and subsequently hired a consultant to assist her. Although she drew heavily upon the practical experience of the consultant to fill in the gaps of her knowledge, she also relied on her firm "no nonsense" approach and her intricate (if newly acquired) knowledge of the organization to ensure that the program was rapidly and appropriately implemented.

"A" then called upon a consultant to provide an external review. The review proved to her CEO (and potentially to regulators) that the backbone of the compliance system was in place with appropriate compliance procedures having been developed. "A" proposes to use her success in this area as a springboard for her own goals and objectives to be promoted within the organization or, alternately, to increase her marketability elsewhere.

The Blue-Collar Leader. "B" was an employee of more than 15 years' standing with the organization and was an excellent blue-collar worker on the front line. "B" was a "legend" inside the organization for his ability to do his job and quite infamous for his flamboyant social life. Everyone had a story of how "B" was a real practical joker, but nevertheless would never let the company down. Further, "B" was also legendary as a workplace health and safety manager for having saved some employees' lives and many others from injury. Although anything but a captive of the company, "B" was nevertheless widely regarded as someone who could always be relied upon to have the appropriate organizational interests at heart.

A major compliance problem appeared in the company requiring detailed technical understanding of the law to assist in the development, articulation, and training of front line employees on some trade practices (antitrust matters). The CEO asked "B" to assist because of how highly he was regarded by these front line employees in the workplace. Previous attempts by internal and external legal counsel to address these concerns had failed badly.

"B," although surprised in being selected, saw the possibilities this appointment would have to assist the company and his own career, and thus took on the assignment with enthusiasm. The CEO advised employees of "B's" appointment and his task, and asked them to help him in developing the best operational solution. "B" sought out and received intensive short-term training on the subject area from internal legal counsel and then, with the assistance of the compliance officer, proposed some draft operational procedures.

"B" convened meetings with local front line employees to discuss the problems and then fine-tuned the draft procedures by himself after these meetings. After having obtained an "in principle" sign off from the internal legal counsel, he then met with a pilot group of front line employees to ascertain whether his solution would work in practice. It was warmly received. "Finally management is listening to one of us," one employee said. The final form of the operational procedure was then signed off by the internal legal counsel and implemented successfully.

The Quiet Achiever. "C" was an internal attorney with the company and was charged with the responsibility of assisting, in conjunction with a project team, with the implementation of regulations stemming from new legislation. The project team included a compliance officer, but "C" was not and did not become the official compliance manager for the project.

"C" had been with the company for more than 10 years and knew the company from the inside as well as anyone. She was an excellent attorney and also understood the new legislation very well. Although quiet and re-tiring by nature, she had excellent interpersonal skills and was an informal source of information and advice to many within the company. During the project "C" introduced many significant compliance systems and reforms and undertook and implemented many product and compliance reviews. She effectively became a mini-compliance professional for many parts of the project.

"C" never appeared on a compliance operational chart, nor did she see herself as a compliance professional. "C" derived no extra kudos or ad-vancement because of her role. After the project was successfully imple-mented, the project team was disbanded and "C" happily returned to her other, full-time legal tasks. Many, if not most, persons inside the company would not have been aware of her massive contribution to the project, nor of her effectiveness in compliance. Indeed, even on the project team, many were not aware of the significant extent of her involvement.

The Traffic Cop. "D" had been with the company for more than 30 years and had watched the company change from one organizational form to another and increase its technological development, sophistication, market share, and geographic spread. "D" had an engineering background and ini-tially worked in the delivery end of the business, but some 12 years ago was made its compliance officer (although he is still referred to as a con-sulting engineer). Without any training in compliance, he presided over the development and implementation of a sophisticated and effective compli-ance system, which was impressive in its results although (perhaps unusu-ally) not officially or formally recognized for these results internally. As one employee said, "That's just the way we do things around here. 'D' has always had a good handle on [compliance] and now his group continues the service."

"D" does not appear on any internal chart as a compliance officer or manager, nor is he seen as a member of the senior executive team. However, he is paid as well as any senior executive and no major decision, even at the board level, is made without checking with "D" as to its possible implications. From an informal perspective, "D" is consulted by many within the organization on a wide range of matters, many of which have nothing to do with compliance. "D" is getting close to retirement and over the years has put in place a comprehensive succession plan. He has also trained a large number of executives in his ways and now finds many of them in senior positions in his and other companies. "D" is somewhat nonplussed by the growing attention he receives, and wants simply to continue "doing the job." But, he does not find it unusual to receive telephone calls from senior members of the government, senior executives of the company, or front line employees of the organization.

"D" has essentially become a "traffic cop," referring problems, solutions, and information to the appropriate persons within the organization. However, when someone even hinted at not following his advice, "D" was able, through subtle (and sometimes not so subtle!) persuasion, to ensure that senior management appropriately reviewed the decision. The "traffic cop" can be blunt and use power when it is required.

COMMON COMPLIANCE PROFESSIONAL ATTRIBUTES

The four compliance professionals described in the previous section exhibited a significant difference in a number of attributes and characteristics. For example, they differed in their self-perception, promotional prospects and aspirations, personal styles and motivations, reputations for "niceness," and remuneration levels. However, they also had many characteristics in common as they sought to deal with the politics of compliance and hence, the "Goals v. Conduct Matrix" described in Figure 14–1.

Two further points need to be made. First, each of these compliance professionals elevated their job descriptions to that of a practitioner of a genuine profession. They each had a sense of vocation, independence, and service based on external norms and expectations that are indicative of a professional rather than an employee. Second, in the manner they practiced their profession, they sought to be cognizant of the "Goals v. Conduct Matrix" referred to in Figure 14–1. Further, in their *style* of practice they sought to use this matrix for the organization's compliance benefit; for example, they seemed to be able to speak in terms of and harness an individual's objectives and goals to achieve compliance-enhancing outcomes. They also shared the following commonalties.

An Authentic Style. Each of the compliance professionals had an authentic style or approach to performing their compliance tasks, and their politicking suited their particular personality. Some were autocratic; some consultative. Some were "nice"; some were tough. Some used power all the time; some used it rarely. But in all instances they used the approach that not only suited them best personally, but also that suited their organization's expectations. In other words, each personal style was successful because it suited the particular organizational corporate culture in general and the compliance culture in particular.

Respect. Whether "high flier" or "floor walker," these compliance professionals enjoyed respect at both the "top" and "bottom" of their organizations. That respect clustered around three core attributes, namely, (1) their personal integrity, (2) their determination to be technically competent and achieve their goals, and (3) their reputations for having the best interests of the organization at heart. Significantly, "B" and "C" had at one time in their careers suffered a loss of status in their companies because they did what they thought was right and in the best interest of the company even though their actions were not in the perceived short-term interests of the organization. Paradoxically, it is this very characteristic that made for their later success in the compliance field. Thus, again reflecting upon the "Goals v. Conduct Matrix," the compliance professionals were "tuned into" key organizational goals and objectives—even in some circumstances when their immediate operational supervisors did not share this view, at least in the short term.

Interpersonal Skills. All the compliance professionals had excellent interpersonal skills and could clearly communicate to and on all levels of their organizations. Although their degree of "niceness" varied, they were always respected and could, when warranted, be extremely tough. Nevertheless, on those occasions when they had to be tough, they also had the ability to make wise and demonstrably fair decisions.

They also seemed to be able to work well with employees and management who were either cynical or altruistic to the point of being naïve. They were able to extract "mileage" from or enlist the support of the most cynical and direct the most naïve in productive ways. And both types of employees were subtly left a bit more in touch with the real organizational goals and objectives of the company. Thus, they also were excellent teachers and trainers, although some had no professional qualifications in these areas. All also seemed to be able to exert a significant degree of personal influence without having to use derived power from the organization, that is, power that was based solely on their organizational position. This is a sign of an expert politician.

Strong Connections in the Organization. All of the compliance professionals knew their organizations intimately and were cognizant of their organization's goals and objectives no matter whether they were public, private, or "real but hidden." These compliance professionals also knew the future direction of the organization, and they understood and were able to "tap into" the fact that this future was known to be "pro compliance." They could thus "add value" to the employee or manager who sought or needed the compliance professional's help by linking compliance and operational advice. There were no "Doctor No's" here, telling people only what *not* to do. They helped people do their jobs well and comply at the same time.

Moreover, there was a real sense of organizational alignment or focus provided by these compliance professionals as they tapped into this future vision, and their existing contacts within the organization and its strategic partners and advisors. Although "B," "C," and "D" had been with their organizations a long time, "A" had not. Yet "A" still had an ability to harness quickly the organizational objectives and establish the internal and external connections needed. It may be easier if compliance professionals, before being appointed, have been with the organization a long time and, importantly, that they know "where the corporate bodies are buried." Nevertheless, newcomers to the task are not disqualified on this ground provided, like "A," that they make the necessary efforts to learn the company quickly and gain the respect needed to work effectively within it. Further, they may strengthen their compliance weaknesses by the use of consultants.

CONCLUSION

A central plank in the practice of compliance remains the ability to manage organizational and individual conduct successfully, and this requires the compliance professional to be an excellent politician in the conflicting organizational and individual goals and objectives discussed in this chapter. This is a key requirement, if not *the* key requirement, for success.

Somewhat paradoxically, however, this ability in politics must not only be an authentic one that matches the professional's personality and attributes, but also must fit neatly into the organizational and compliance cultures in which the compliance professional seeks to serve.

NOTES

1. R. Dennings, Compliance from Scratch: Step-by-Step Designed Implementation and Evaluation (unpublished manuscript; on file with author).
2. *See* Figure 14–1.
3. For further information on the difference between behavioral and procedural aspects of compliance, see B. Dee, *Characterising Conduct as "Behavioural" or "Procedural,"* 5 Compliance News (1998).
4. *See* Figure 14–1.
5. For a formal list of ideal characteristics of the successful compliance professional, see the *Australian Standard on Compliance Programs*, Standards Australia AS3806. Clause 3.2.4. states:

    The senior executive responsible for overseeing compliance should have direct access to the Chief Executive Officer and any audit or compliance committee.

    The senior executive or, where employed, compliance manager should:

    (a) have a high status, authority, recognition and support within the organization;

    (b) have a record of integrity and commitment to compliance;

    (c) have access to expert knowledge of relevant laws, regulations, codes and organizational standards;

    (d) have good communication skills;

    (e) have access to staff or advisors who are able to translate legal and other compliance obligations into everyday organizational procedures;

    (f) be responsible for ensuring that practices and documentation comply with the law, including ensuring that such obligations are understood and observed by relevant managers and staff;

    (g) have access to all levels of the organization, as necessary, to ensure compliance;

    (h) be able to consider and advise on compliance problems encountered by staff;

    (i) be both a formal and informal reference point on compliance matters;

    (j) be responsible for the overall design, consistency and integrity of the system; and

    (k) have access to senior decision makers and participate in the organization's senior decision-making process.

    In order to perform their duties effectively, staff need access to material resources that may include:

    1. detailed manuals on compliance procedures, reference material and database;

    2. adequate work tools and facilities; and

    3. internal and external support mechanisms and networks (e.g., staff newsletters).

Index

A

Access
  audit committee, 140
  chief executive officer, 140
  compliance program
    personnel, 142–143
    records, 143
  empowerment, 140
Accreditation, profession, 5
Antitrust Division's Corporate
  Leniency Program, 149
Attorney, 26–28
  compliance program, 142–143
  conflict of interest, 109
Audit committee, access, 140
Auditing, 38, 44, 68
Authority, 138
  corporate ethics and compliance
    officer, 218–219
Autonomy, profession, 2, 3–4

B

Benchmarking, 69

Best practices, 67
Bioethics
  compliance, contrasted,
    171–173
  dialysis "God squad," 170
  historical overview, 169–171
Biomedical model
  characterized, 158–159
  organizational ethics, 158–159
Biomedicine, atomistic
  foundationalism, 168–169
Blue collar leader, compliance,
  273–274
Board of directors
  compliance program resolution,
    138–139, 152–153
  reporting, 138–139
Body of knowledge, bureaucrat,
  174
Boredom, 197, 202–203
Bribery, 95–96
Bureaucrat
  body of knowledge, 174
  health care compliance
    professional, 174